The Busy Body Fitness Manual

A FIFTEEN MINUTES A DAY EXERCISE PROGRAMME FOR BUSY PEOPLE

Pamela Carsaniga

Illustrations by James Starey

ALLEN & UNWIN

First published in 1996 by
Allen & Unwin Pty Ltd
9 Atchinson Street, St Leonards, NSW 2065 Australia
Phone: (61 2) 9901 4088
Fax: (61 2) 9906 2218
E-mail: 100252.103@compuserve.com

National Library of Australia
Cataloguing-in-Publication entry:

Carsaniga, Pamela.
The busy body fitness manual: a fifteen minute a day exercise programme for busy people.

ISBN 1 86448 133 1.

1. Exercise - Handbooks, manuals, etc. 2. Physical fitness - Handbooks, manuals, etc. I. Title.

613.71

Designed by Seymour Design
Set in 12/15pt Garamond 3
10 9 8 7 6 5 4 3 2 1

Contents

Standing sequences

Floor sequences

Foreword

At last an effective exercise plan I can confidently take on board without qualms! Fitness is a number one priority for actors, yet our irregular day to day living means that a routine is out of the question except for brief and usually unexpected periods. An actor needs to adapt to constantly varying demands, long hours in rehearsal or on the set, travelling and setting up home in new surroundings or staying in hotels.

In this often challenging, occasionally satisfying, sometimes exciting or frustrating lifestyle it's essential to minimise stress. My experience has proved that regular exercise offers the best antidote to stress, but for weeks at a time it may be impossible to fit a workout into a day's schedule. When I do have a couple of hours to myself, I like to spend time with family and friends or to read. This fifteen minute a day plan is the answer for me. Wherever I am, I can fit a session in and be confident that I'm maintaining a level of physical fitness that prepares me to front up to a performance or a game of tennis.

The principles underlying the exercises are recognisably drawn from those time-honoured techniques of Laban and Alexander, based on good posture and safe movement practices. Pamela Carsaniga's instructions are simple to follow. A glance at James Starey's zany illustrations is enough to prompt the memory after working through a sequence a few times. I usually select five or six of the sequences to do at a session; I find that's sufficient to leave me feeling invigorated yet calm. The combination of movement, stretch and relaxation reduces tension and stress immediately, and a few weeks of the programme has built up my strength and flexibility. I confidently recommend it to people of either sex and any age.

GRETA SCACCHI

Introduction

THE FACTS

Medical research findings, as the media persistently reports, point to physical exercise as a crucial factor in maintaining overall health and wellbeing. Recently published statistics suggest that regular exercise results in an actual increase in bone density, even in people of advanced age. Faced with this kind of evidence few would deny the need to actively engage in an exercise programme — a need that has become more imperative in a society which travels mainly on wheels, and where walking in cities and suburbs is more of a health hazard than a pleasure. Improved posture and balance, flexibility and mobility are further benefits to be gained from exercises conceived with a focus on good body alignment and rational application of effort.

THE DAY TO DAY REALITY

The path to maintaining physical fitness and a well-toned body is strewn with brave attempts, abandoned initiatives and relinquished objectives. The reason for this is easy to see: if you wish to stick to any of the many forms of exercise or physical workouts available (and there are several which are highly commendable in various city and suburban locations) you need not only constant discipline, but a considerable outlay of time, money and effort. Add to an hour spent on aerobics, yoga, Alexander, Pilates or working out at the gym the time it takes getting to and from the venue, the outlay of cash, plus the strain of fitting in with a busy schedule. For some of us, succumbing to the demands of family or the pressures of work becomes easier than adhering to regular attendance at the gym.

A PERSONAL CASE

When I decided I could no longer ignore the need for a regular exercise schedule, my personal difficulty was finding a suitable one. A background in dance training and in safe movement practice made me reject aerobics. I believed I was equipped with the know-how to arrange a more effective exercise programme for myself but I lacked the time, the discipline and the space to establish a regular habit when there were always other tasks competing for priority. Weeks drifted into months and, as the months became years, the lack of purposeful exercise began to make its mark, firstly in my general wellbeing — both physical and psychological — and then in my appearance.

That's when I resolved to attempt to regain fitness with a fifteen minute session a day. Fifteen minutes a day would be a great improvement on no exercise at all and it was an amount of time I could realistically aim to fit in between other commitments.

In fact my regular fifteen minute slot turned out to be more beneficial than two one-hourly sessions a week. The result was so positive that my daughter asked me to write my programme out for her. I realised that there would be many others who might enjoy it, like the groups for whom, some years ago, I had prepared a weekly workout based on modern dance exercises. Remembering the positive feedback I'd had from them encouraged me to produce this volume.

THE FLY IN THE OINTMENT

The movements need to be approached with attention to detail to be effective. In the initial stages your fifteen minutes will be spent grasping the basic features of each movement and establishing beneficial and safe habits. A positive aspect here, especially for the novice exerciser, is that by studying the preparatory positions and gradually following through perhaps two or three sequences a day, there will be little risk of straining unaccustomed body parts. The initial inconvenience will prove a long-term advantage in preventing overexertion at one session.

The basic exercise principles explained in the manual must be understood and put into practice in the separate components. These components are then combined in brief movement sequences to promote an increased energy level through varied activity. A couple of weeks' regular application should provide a functional set of exercises: by the end of the first month the benefits will be evident.

BUSY BODY BENEFITS

Whatever your routine, whether it be a concentrated session at the computer, coping with the kids, an overlong stint at the workbench or a trip to the supermarket, a fifteen minute break will help to restore a balanced perspective. It will enable you to take stock and consider how you are treating yourself both physically and mentally. The revitalising effect will more than make up for the time spent. Shop assistants and bank clerks, constantly travelling executives, flight attendants with irregular lifestyles, fulltime parents, anyone who can find a space roughly three by three metres can embark on this plan with an outlay of just fifteen minutes a day. For people who are too busy or unable to attend exercise classes, have no taste for it or are simply interested in an alternative, this programme will:

* Improve posture through correct body alignment.

* Improve muscle tone.

* Encourage beneficial movement habits in normal everyday activities.

* Help to get back into condition after a break.

* Serve as a quick revitaliser at any time of the day.

THE CHOICE IS YOURS

This fifteen minute a day plan comprises several alternative sessions. Which you choose to do depends on your immediate need. If you have just got up from a sedentary task you may want to get your whole body moving with the introductory 'sway' sequence followed by the 'reach and roll'. If you are taking a break from being on your feet, or want to re-energise before preparing for an evening out, you may want to begin by lying flat on your back to loosen and relax, and finish up with the 'reach and roll'. The exercises can be mixed as desired, with the proviso that a cat-like stretch followed by a sequence involving large muscle groups is recommended for an initial warm-up.

Each sequence has an in-built rhythmic flow which helps to sustain the energy level. The relative time counts are shown and can be applied as the sequence is mastered. Some people, however, find greater stimulation in exercising to music. In line with my personal preference for 1940s style jazz, and especially for such greats as Louis Armstrong and Thomas 'Fats' Waller, appropriate suggestions are listed at the end of the book. These would also indicate the envisaged pace of the sequences when the components are combined. If you wish to put the sequences to your own musical preferences, ensure you use a tempo and rhythm that allows and encourages you to stretch, control, relax and use gravity as each exercise requires.

The illustrations will provide a quick visual cue once the movements are understood as well as backing up the verbal explanations. James Starey designed the clownish character specifically to emphasise the premise of *The Busy Body Fitness Manual*, that the programme has no age or gender bias. The plan is designed so that you work at your own personal level and, providing you apply the basic principles, you will obtain the benefits.

Approaching the programme

The programme is structured on brief sequences, each comprising several movements to give variety and create flow. This will maximise the benefit for the precious time and effort expended and should also stimulate a feeling of wellbeing. By combining various movements into a sequence, we avoid the strain that can result from repetitive concentration on an isolated body part. Embarking on such a movement programme requires some initial learning. For each exercise you need to fully understand the basic principles in order to form beneficial habits; you need to become familiar with the sequence and to apply efforts at the appropriate points while maintaining the dynamic flow. These different facets are interdependent: you apply effort in accordance with the basic principles, within the context of the sequence; the tempo counts create a dynamic flow with a natural breathing pattern — but where to begin? Start from the separate components, then work out the sequence, check the relative basic principles and gradually apply more effort as you master the movements and learn where you should focus to achieve maximum benefit. Accordingly, the programme:

* introduces the components;
* explains the movement sequence with time counts;
* outlines the basic principles and general comments or special points; and
* suggests further developments and alternatives.

It is essential to know *how* to execute a movement. To ensure clarity and accuracy, explanations sometimes need to be lengthy. Once the basics are grasped, however, headings and illustrations should suffice as a reminder. In large aerobics classes where time is too limited to allow for individual supervision, people may imitate an instructor without applying the essential techniques. You won't have this problem! Take time to execute each component separately and precisely to enable your body to fully experience the desired effect, then link them in the sequence. This will have an indirect benefit: it will prevent excessive exercise in the early stages and avoid painful muscles the next day. Start gently and proceed to a more vigorous level especially if you are just beginning or are out of practice. Once you have assimilated the basic principles, you can go directly to the outlined sequence with confidence. However, even when you have become familiar with a sequence, it's a good idea to return occasionally and check the points to ensure you are not glossing over an important aspect.

Throughout the manual, we suggest some alternative sequences to diversify and enlarge on the basic movements. Doubtless you will add your own once the principles are mastered.

Enjoy the programme!

TECHNICAL NOTE

Some movements specify your feet should be 'turned out' and others require 'parallel feet'. The terms refer to the angle of the feet in relation to the body. When standing with your feet together in 'turn out', your heels are touching and your toes are apart. Always adopt a degree of turn out which feels easy. This position is more natural for sideways movements such as the initial 'sway'. In actual fact your whole legs should be 'turned out' to avoid twisting joints: your knees will always face the same direction as your feet.

The same applies for the term 'feet parallel' where the inside line of one foot, from big toe to heel, is parallel to the other and your toes are pointing directly forward. This position helps to make you more aware of the direction of feet, knees and also of hips and helps achieve stability in movements which involve isolated body parts.

The distance between your feet will naturally relate to individual stature.

The term 'centre' refers to an imaginary plumb line dropped from the crown of the head and finishing between the feet. It is a useful mental image to hold on to for standing sequences and is used in the floor sequences where the imaginary line will, of course, be horizontal but retain the same body relationship.

Special note regarding 'mirror image' illustrations

For sideways movements which occur in several sequences, the illustrative character is shown facing you in the manner of a class instructor. This means that although the boxed instructions may say, for example, 'sway to your right', the model is swaying left. This mirror image has been adopted to make the exercises easier to follow. Where a movement is repeated several times within a sequence, the model will show only the first movement to each side. The number of repeats are suggested in the boxed instructions.

Standing SEQUENCES

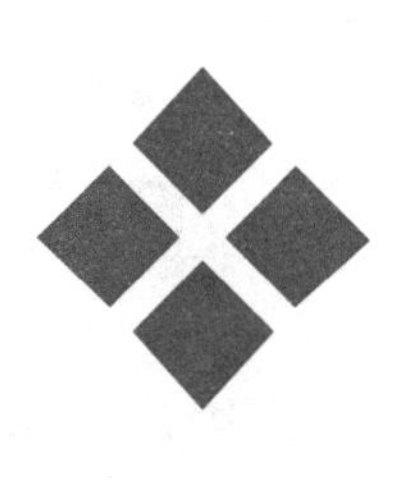

1 *Pendulum sways: an overall warm-up*

The aim of this first exercise is to involve the whole body in movements to stimulate breathing and circulation. As you warm up and lubricate the joints, the sensation of movement invariably has a tonic effect on mood as well as on physique. If you were tempted to convince yourself that today you really didn't have the energy to embark on your fifteen minute programme, this exercise will alter your perspective and restore vitality.

The sway is set up by transferring your weight from one foot to the other with an easy rock. Place your feet in a natural turn out; the distance between them will be about two of your feet lengths apart but this may increase as the sway gathers momentum. Allow your knees to bend as you pass through the central position and to straighten as you transfer your weight on to one leg. Gradually increase the depth of the knee bend as you make the transfer, and at the same time increase the lean in your torso and let your arms swing across in pendulum fashion. Make use of your body weight by giving in to gravity for both knee bends and arm swings.

Introduction to pendulum sways

Stand comfortably with your feet apart in a natural turn out and your weight evenly distributed between them.

Flex your knees slightly, then transfer your weight onto one foot, straightening both knees.

& 1

Return to your central starting position, flexing your knees, then transfer your weight onto the other foot in the same way.

& 2

Repeat, making a swaying movement from side to side and allowing the arms to swing pendulum fashion, parallel to each other, across your body.

Recommended time counts are in **BOLD**.

Remember...:

❖ Let your arms relax and feel heavy and long; allow gravity to operate as they drop and resist it as you reach to the side.

❖ Gradually let your torso follow your arms into an easy sideways lean.

❖ As the sway gathers momentum, think of fully stretching the ankle as you take your weight off it.

❖ Give in to gravity for an easier knee bend, and feel your breath flowing easily.

❖ Check that the degree of your feet turn-out is the same as your thighs so that your flexed knee is directly over your toe.

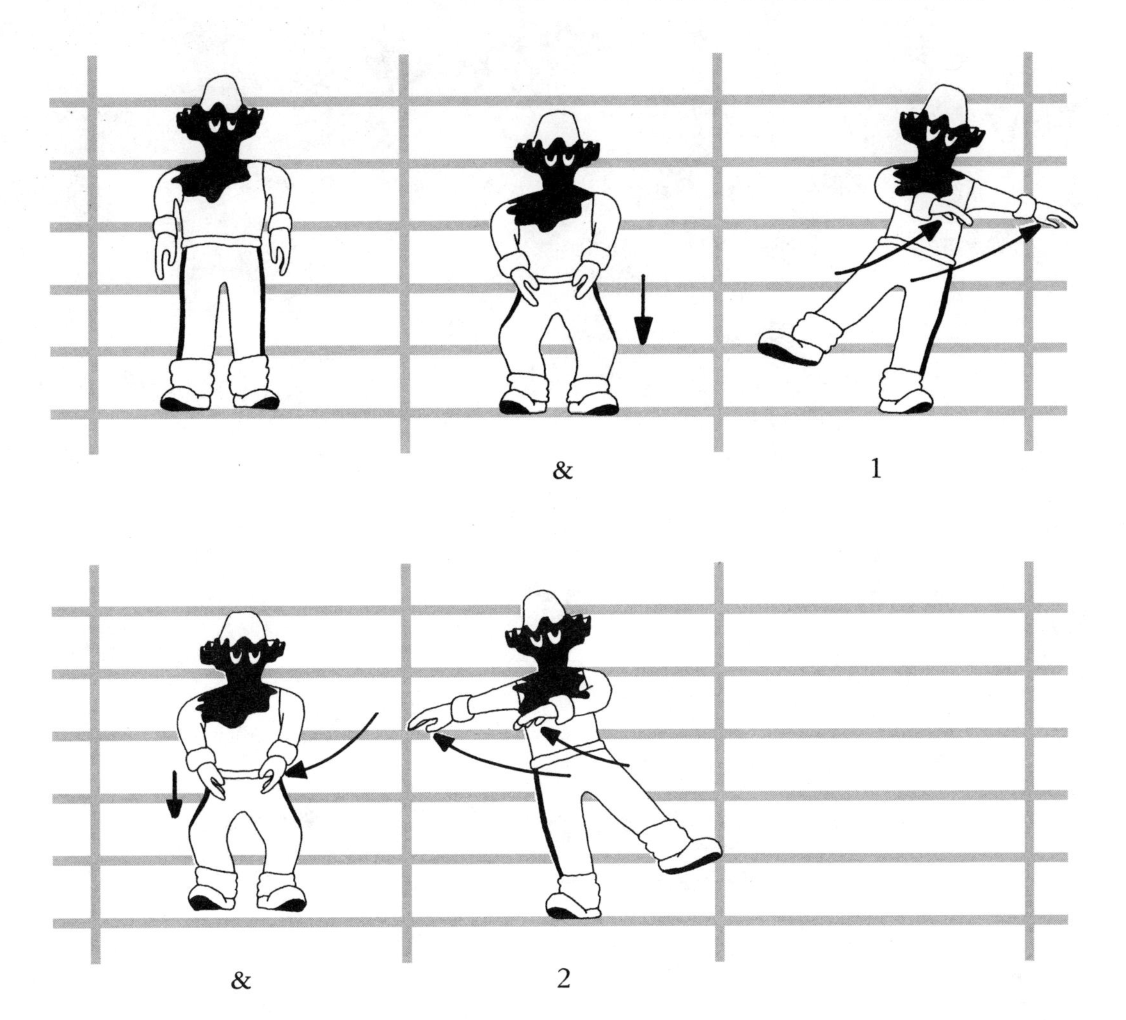
&
1
&
2

Side to side with parallel arm circling

Sway sideways to your right, swinging parallel arms to the right.

& 1

Sway sideways left, swinging parallel arms to the left.

& 2

Sway sideways right, close left foot to right rising onto balls of the feet, circling parallel arms from the right to over the head and down.

& 3

Step sideways right into a sway again, swinging parallel arms to the right.

& 4

Repeat on the other side.

Remember:

❖ Make easy, relaxed movements to begin.

❖ Your feet will probably be about the length of two feet apart. Bend your knees as far as is comfortable without bending the torso forwards; the depth of your knee bend should increase as the movement becomes familiar and you gain strength.

❖ Push away from the floor with your foot for extra strength and flexibility.

❖ As your sense of balance grows more confident, let the arms take the torso into a side lean.

❖ When your arms feel long and heavy, gradually introduce more stretch by reaching to the sides and overhead on the circle.

❖ Check that your knee is directly over the line of your foot as you bend. If it is not, adjust your turn out to align them correctly.

❖ Deepen your knee bend as you feel able but keep an easy movement.

❖ When your joints feel warm and supple, increase the force of the ankle stretch as you push away from the floor. Feel the pressure through your foot from toe to heel as you replace your weight on it.

❖ When you are confident in all aspects of the sways and arm circling, you may wish to add a head roll by following your hands with your eyes: your head will then extend the direction of the lean. Circle your head down — chin to the top of the breastbone — on the knee bend, and complete the circle with face looking towards the ceiling as your arms pass overhead.

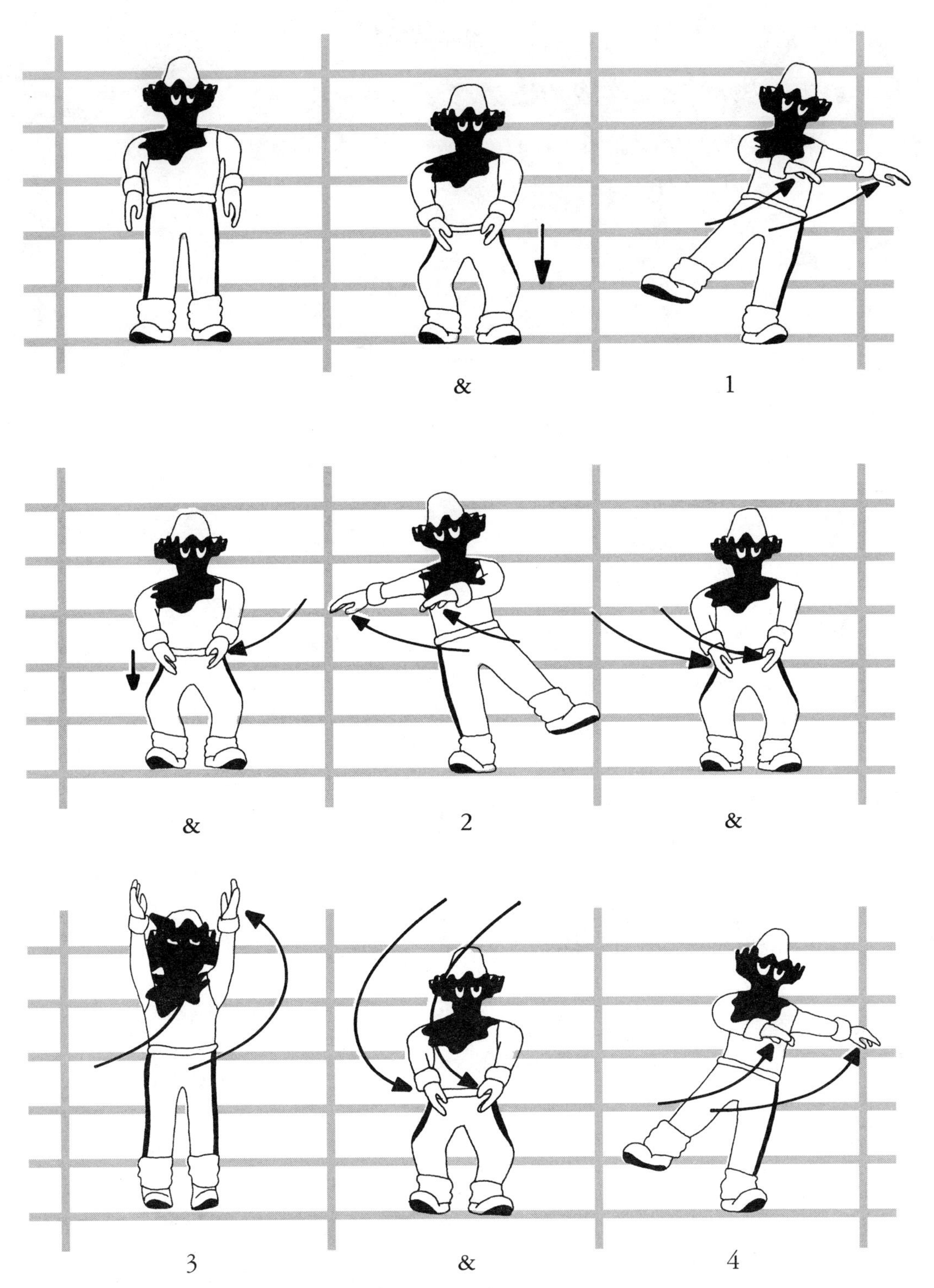

NOTE: These illustrations mirror the instructions

Forward and backward diagonal sways with single arm swings and circle

Step in a forward diagonal left direction with the left foot (using the bending and stretching motion), swinging the right arm along the same line to a forward reach.

& 1

Step diagonally back on the right foot, swinging the right arm down and into a backward reach.

& 2

Step forward left; close right foot to left rising on the balls of the feet; step forward left, making a complete (forward, up, back, down) circle with the right arm to finish in a forward reach.

& 3 & 4

Reverse the combination (stepping back on the right, forward on the left, back on the right, close left to right, step back on the right) with a reverse arm circle (back, up, forward, down) to finish in a backward reach.

& 1–& 4

When you have done the movement a few times on the left side, repeat it with the right foot stepping forward diagonally to the right with the left arm swinging and circling. You can change from one side to the other by inserting a small change step on the & before the count 1.

Remember . . .

❖ Let your shoulders go with the swinging arm in the forward and backward directions so that the torso is turning from the waist.

❖ Encourage the torso to lean along the forward and backward diagonals to involve muscles in adjusting for balance.

❖ Keep the head and neck in an easy and natural line with the torso; the eye direction will be forward and slightly down with the forward step, and back towards the hand on the backward step.

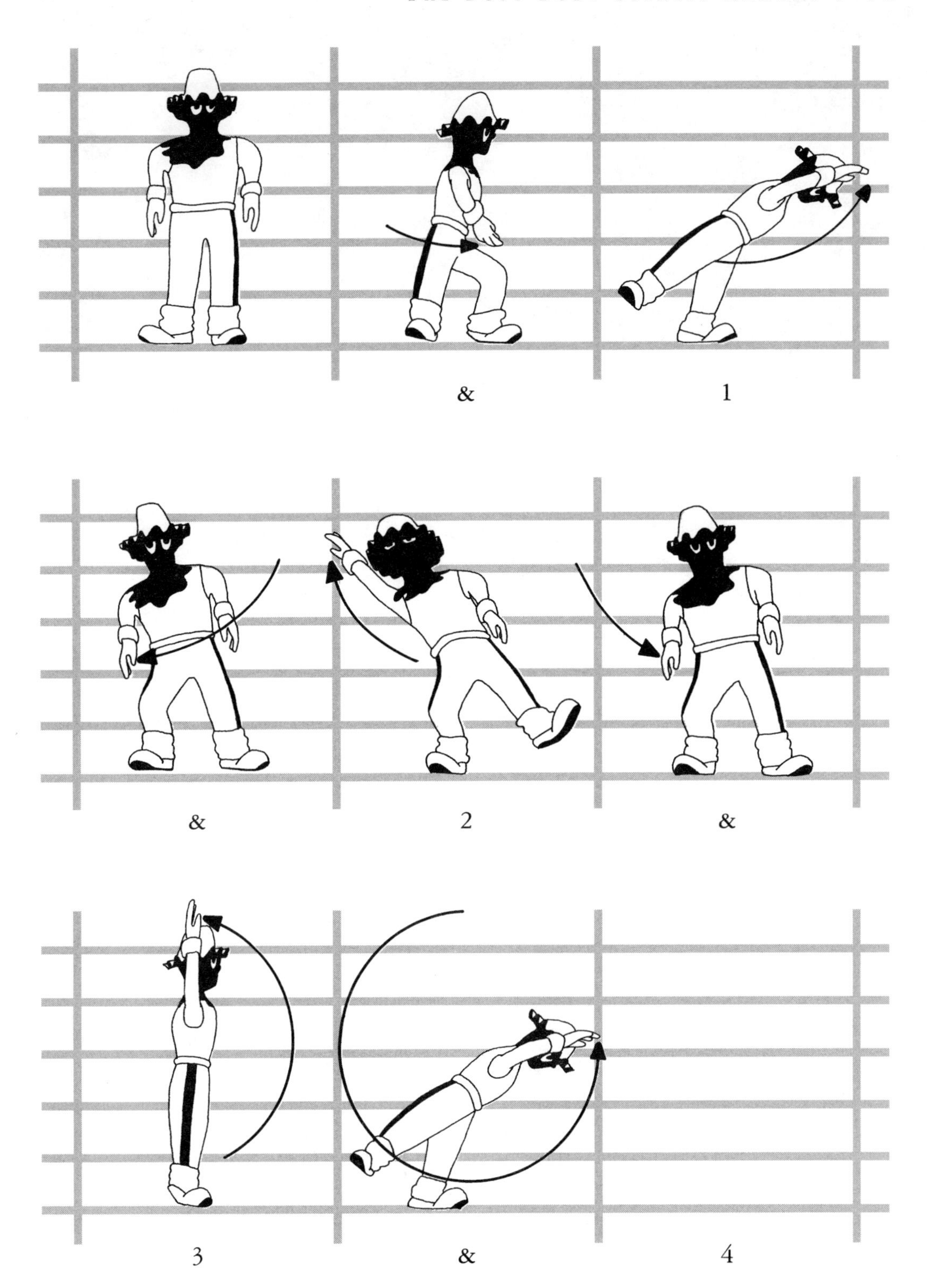
&
1
&
2
&
3
&
4

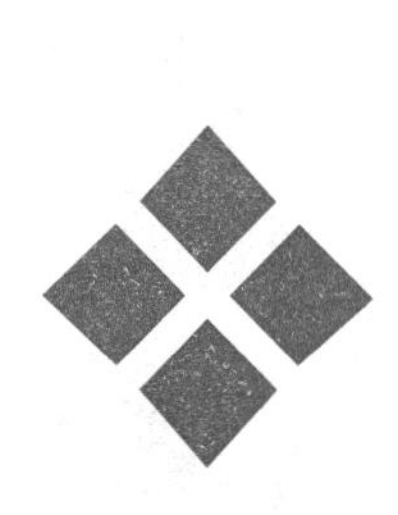

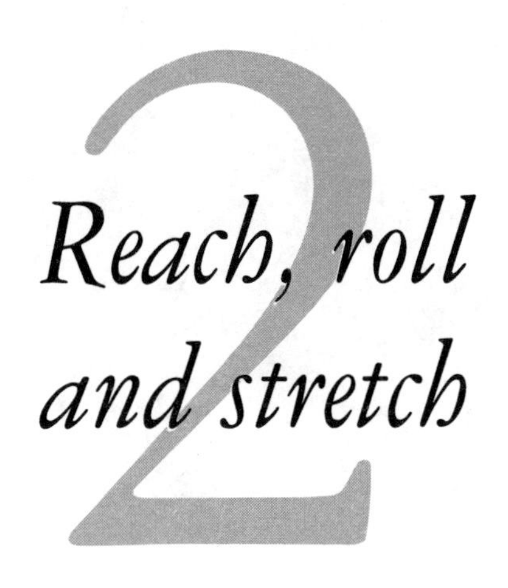

Reach, roll and stretch

PREPARATION FOR THE ROLL

The roll forward and recovery is one of the critical components in an exercise programme because it involves the beneficial use of the spine as well as the abdominal muscles and forms the basis of a good body alignment. The term alignment refers to the setting of the body parts in relation to each other. A tilted pelvis or drooping shoulders can put a strain on the spine. Correct alignment promotes a sense of lightness and vitality. Stand tall and sense the spine as a vertical axis with the head balanced on top. Shoulders and arms are relaxed and hanging, breathing is deep and easy, hips are centred — neither tilted forward or back; feet are parallel, and about the width of your hips apart. In practising the roll consider the head an extension of the spine and use its weight.

Your head leads the roll. Let it drop forward: shoulders will follow as you slowly curve the spine as low as you can go without releasing the hip joint (shoulders remain relaxed so that your arms will hang in front of your legs). At this point allow the knees to bend forward over the toes and, pulling in your lower abdomen (think of pressing your navel in towards the spine), go lower with your head and torso, and hang there to feel the extension across the back of the rib cage due to the weight of hanging arms and relaxed neck. Move your head gently to check the neck is relaxed.

Drop down to place your hands in front of your feet.

Try straightening your knees if you like but, before you begin to unroll your spine, bend your knees slightly forward again and tilt the hips forward (tuck your tail under). Now hold the navel/abdomen in as you come smoothly up and finally re-centre the hips and replace the head on top of the spine. Try this roll several times until you have assimilated all the aspects and then combine it in the following sequence.

Easy top to toe stretch

Standing erect with your feet parallel under your hips, lift your arms above your head and reach high alternately with right and left, twice each.

1–4

Let your arms collapse softly as you drop your head and roll forward.

5–8

Drop your hips to a crouching position and reach forward with your hands near the floor.

&

Transfer your weight partially onto your hands as you straighten and stretch your legs.

1, 2

Return to a crouching position with your hands just in front of your feet.

&

Straighten your legs as far as possible without straining.

3, 4

Bend your knees forward and unroll to stand erect.

5–8

Raise arms again to repeat four times or more.

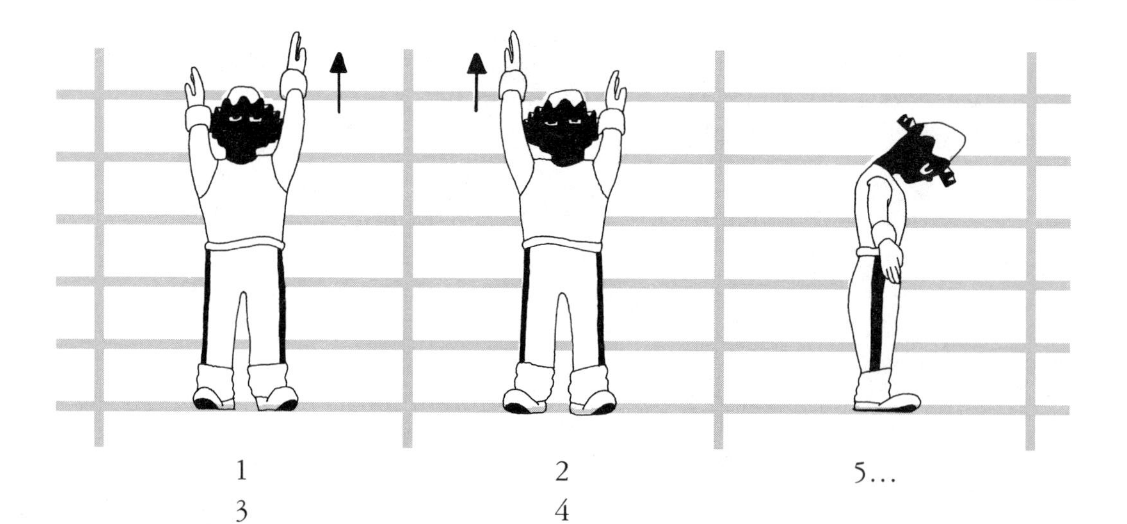

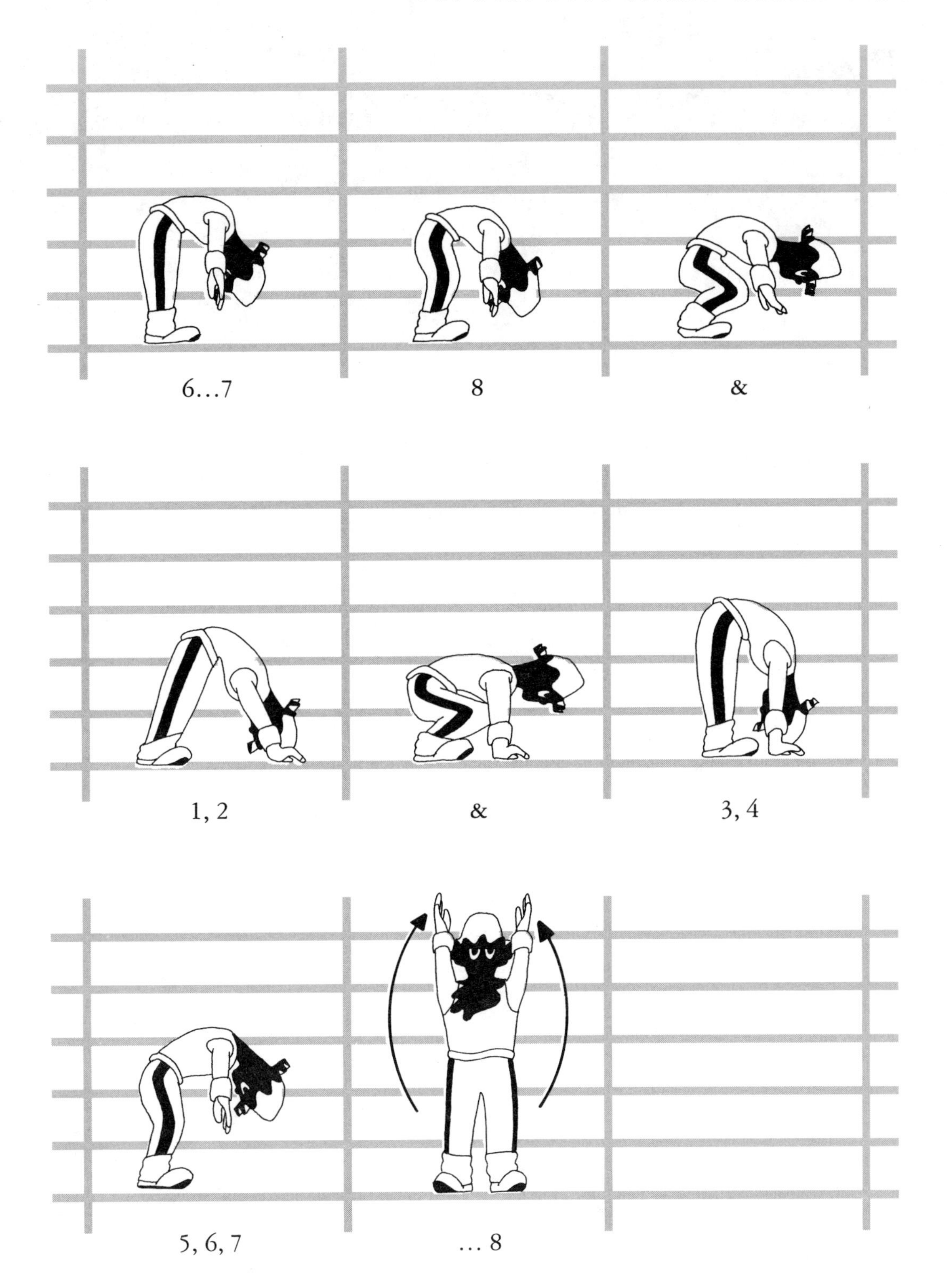
6…7
8
&
1, 2
&
3, 4
5, 6, 7
… 8

Remember:

❖ Reach high with your fingertips so that you feel a full stretch through the side of the body.

❖ Check through the finer points of the roll and recovery to ensure all points are observed and to gain maximum benefit.

❖ On the crouch and leg stretch movements, fold and unfold the joints softly (hip, knee, ankle) to increase flexibility gently and without strain. Ensure your head is down on these stretches to use its weight to advantage.

A FINAL NOTE: It is counterproductive to stretch your hamstrings (back of the leg) to the point of producing pain. If the exercise is done regularly, flexibility will gradually increase, whereas too ambitious stretching at the beginning can cause resistance, tension and possible damage, following which you will have to rest and lose the benefits gained.

The principles outlined in this roll and recovery also represent the most economic and effortless method of getting down onto the floor and more especially for returning to a standing position. By raising your hips with your hands on the floor and head and torso at a low level, less strain is placed on leg joints and muscles.

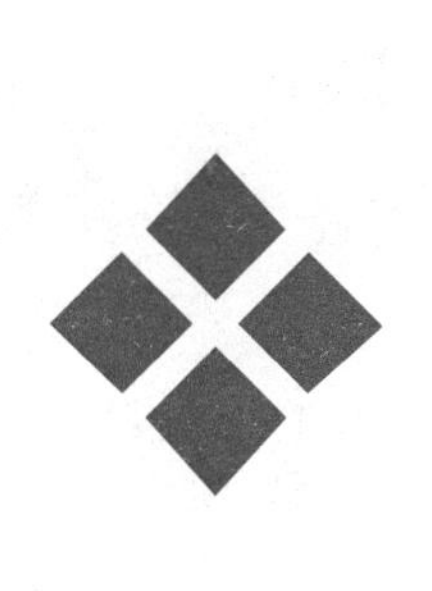

3 *Leg lifts for balance, poise and flexibility*

This simple exercise uses a basic step sequence to give impetus for lifting the leg in the hip socket. As you swing your leg up, maintain a relaxed knee so that you maximise the range of mobility in the hip joint. More flexible people may want to try the same movement with a straight leg once the hip joint is warmed up.

With front lift

Step forward with your right foot.

1

Swing your left knee forward and high.

2

Step back with your left foot.

3

Step back with your right foot.

4

Repeat, beginning with the left foot.

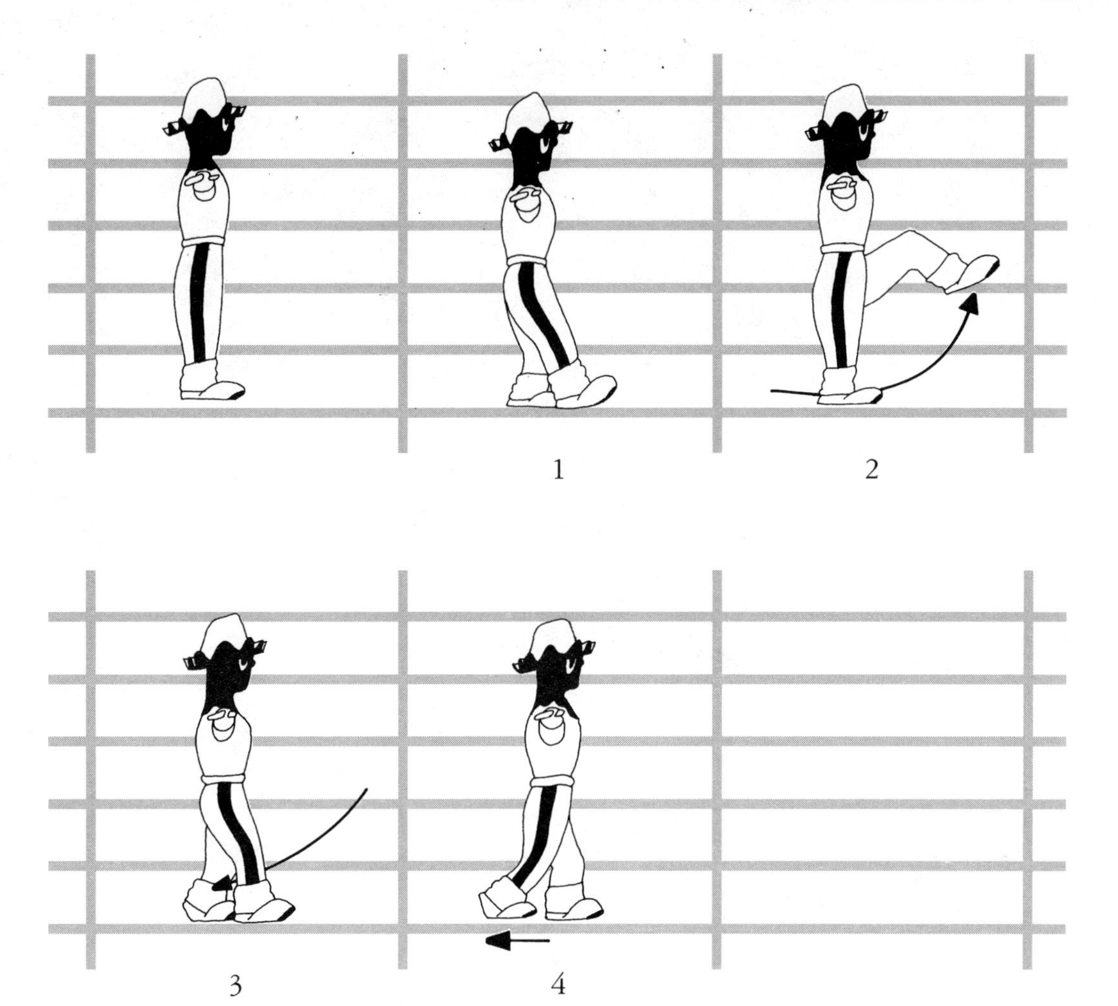
1
2
3
4

With side lift

Use the same basic step sequence.

Step right foot across in front of left.

1

Swing your left knee to the side and high.

2

Step left foot back behind right.

3

Step right foot sideways to the right.

4

Repeat, beginning with the left foot.

Remember:

❖ Use one beat for each movement.

❖ Hold the arms out to the side and slightly in front of you for balance.

❖ Hold the torso and head steady, taking care not to duck down as the leg is lifted. Allow the knee of the supporting leg to stretch and flex normally, as for walking.

❖ You may feel you can use a springy walk with this combination.

❖ You may also like to add an alternative arm gesture to counterbalance the raised leg.

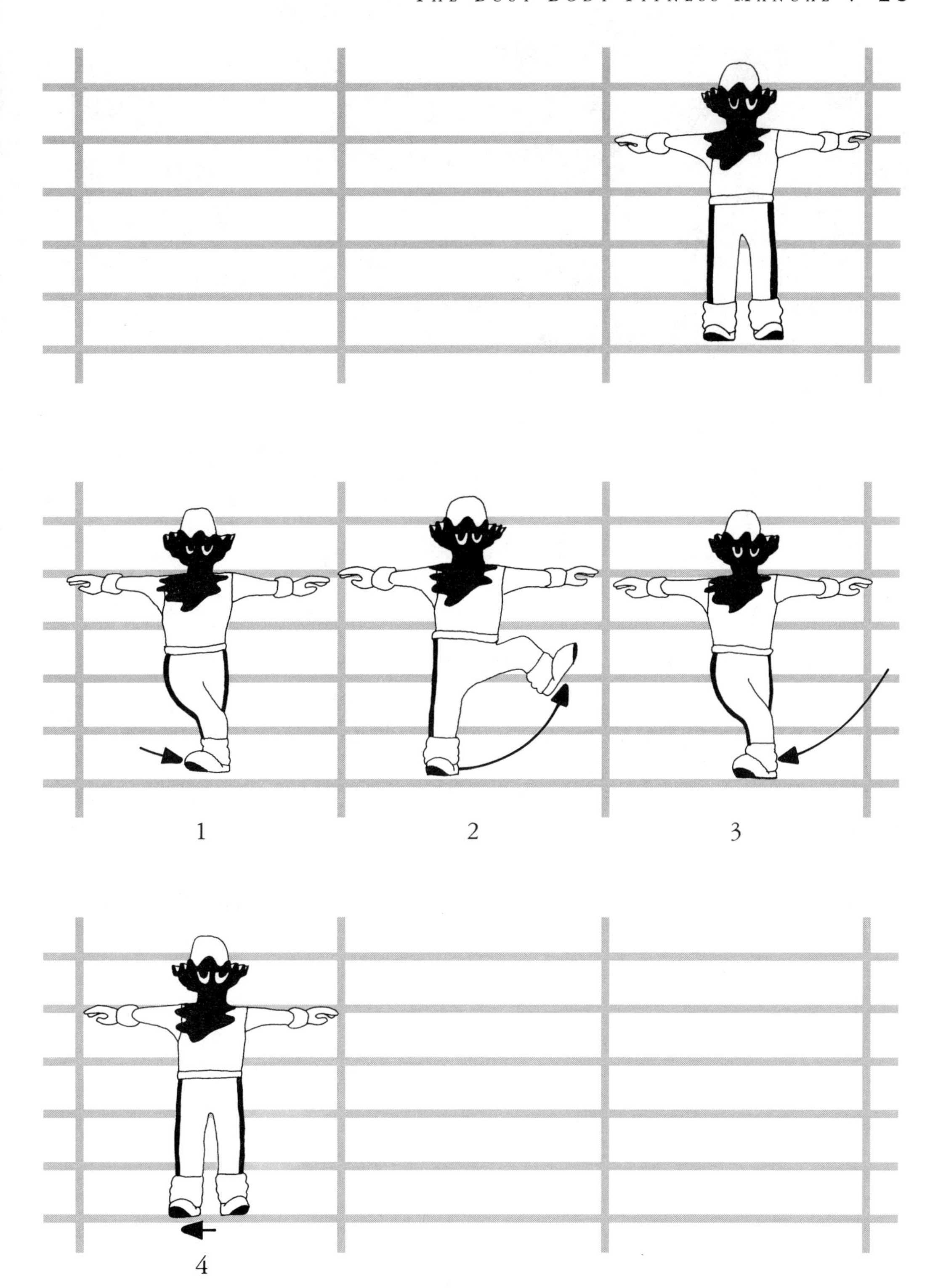
1
2
3
4

With back lift

Use the same basic step sequence.

Step forward right and raise your left leg straight out behind you, bending the knee of the supporting leg and letting your torso come forward as much as necessary.

1, 2

Step back with your left foot.

3

Step back with your right foot.

4

Repeat, beginning with the left foot.

Remember:

❖ The aim here is to strengthen the back and abdomen. Maximum benefit is gained on the backward leg lift if the raised leg is kept well stretched and the abdomen held flat and tight. This is more essential than a high leg.

❖ The arms can be stretched and held slightly away from the body on count 2, and allowed to relax across the body on counts 3–4. This arm movement makes for easier flow and balance.

❖ A combination of four sequences for each direction is suggested to make the exercise continuous and varied.

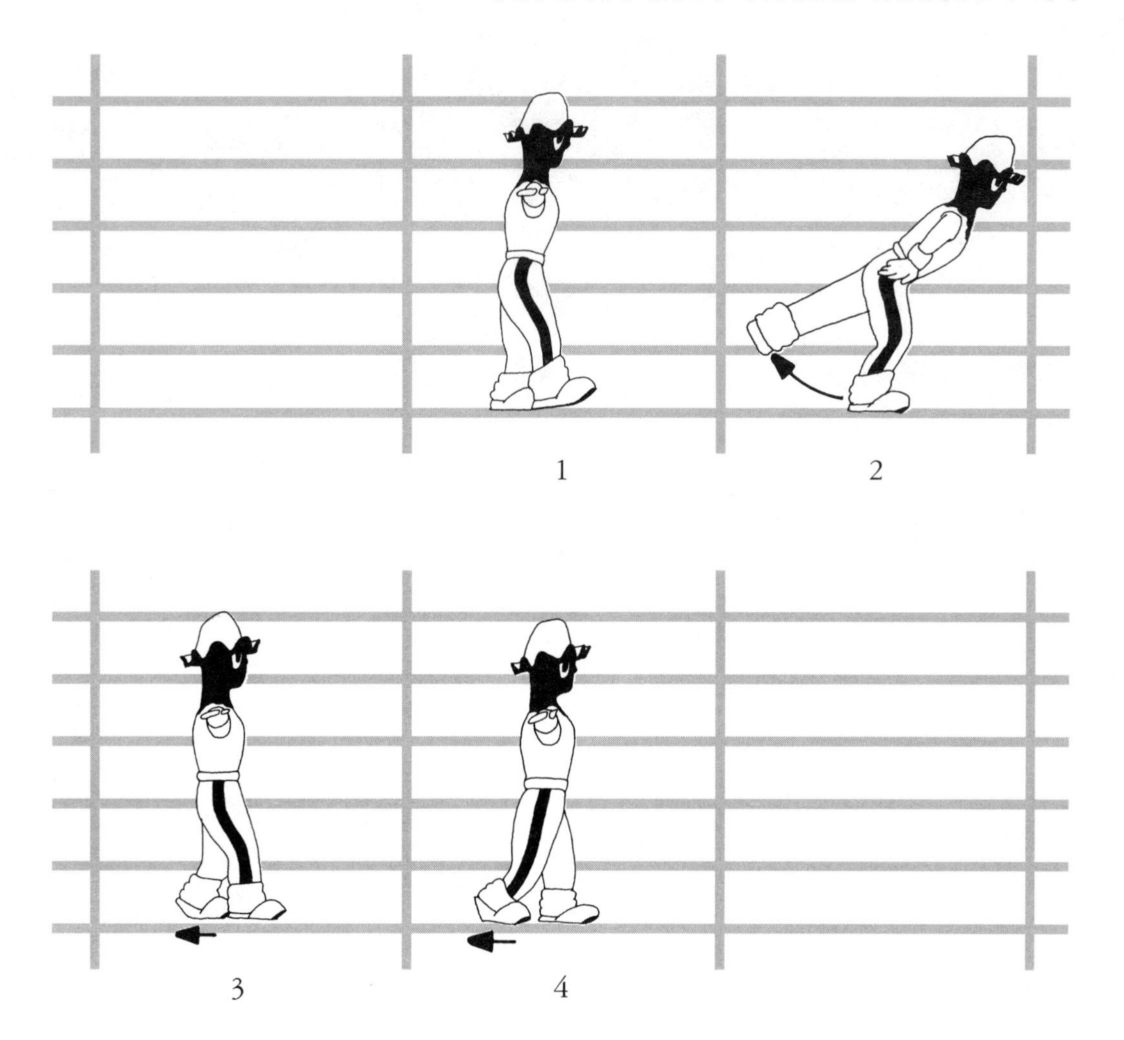
1
2
3
4

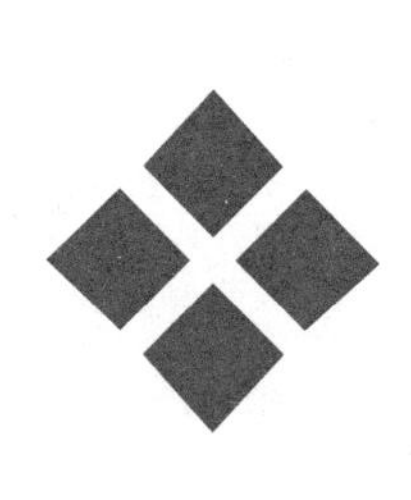

4 *Side bends and rotation for upper torso flexibility*

This sequence works on awareness of line and flexibility in the upper torso, that is the rib-cage area and shoulders. Seasoned exercisers will be able to embark directly on the sequence, but the novice may require a more gradual approach to successfully fulfil the requirements. These movements may feel awkward, since they rarely occur through the limited physical demands of today's lifestyle. Follow the sequence, and then work through it gently, noting the recommendations below. It should not take long to acquire familiarity and to gain the benefit.

For the novice, the side bends will present no difficulty in execution once you have felt the effect of fully stretching the raised arm as you bend (see the illustration).

However, the semicircular path described for the upper spine calls for attention to detail in order to maximise the benefits of the exercise. You may wish to try the pattern of the sequence first with a simple head rotation for the forward movement, and an upwards and slightly backwards reach with your head for the second section. Adding the arm movements will help to define the directions and maintain shoulder joint mobility.

For this sequence, stand tall with feet parallel and with the distance between them equivalent to the width of your hips. You may wish to learn the arm pattern first, then add more vigour to the movement and fully involve the head and upper spine in the circular path.

With forward torso rotation

Swing your fully stretched left arm out sideways, up high and over to the right so that it takes your torso into a side bend. At the same time allow your relaxed right arm to swing in front of you.

& 1

As your left arm retraces its path, swing your right arm out through the side position, up high and over to the left (the left arm swings in front of you).

& 2

Repeat again for each side.

& 3, & 4

Make a fifth swing over to the right with the left arm and follow with a complete circular path in front of you using your upper torso and arms. As the left arm passes the right, the right follows it passing across to your left, up over your head and out to the side.

& 5–& 8

Repeat the first eight counts, beginning by swinging the right arm over to the left.

& 1–& 8

Remember:

❖ Remember that this is not merely an arm movement; it also involves the upper torso.

❖ To achieve the aim of working the upper spine, leave the arms straight (no bent elbows), long and heavy yet at the same time maintain a feeling of reach.

❖ Breathe easily and use the head to extend the side curve.

❖ Check that the side bends stay within the side plane and are not curving either forward or back.

❖ On the circular movement, firmly hold the hips and middle torso in place while you involve the upper back. The head and shoulders move in a half circle from the side, through a forward curve to the other side and return to the erect position.

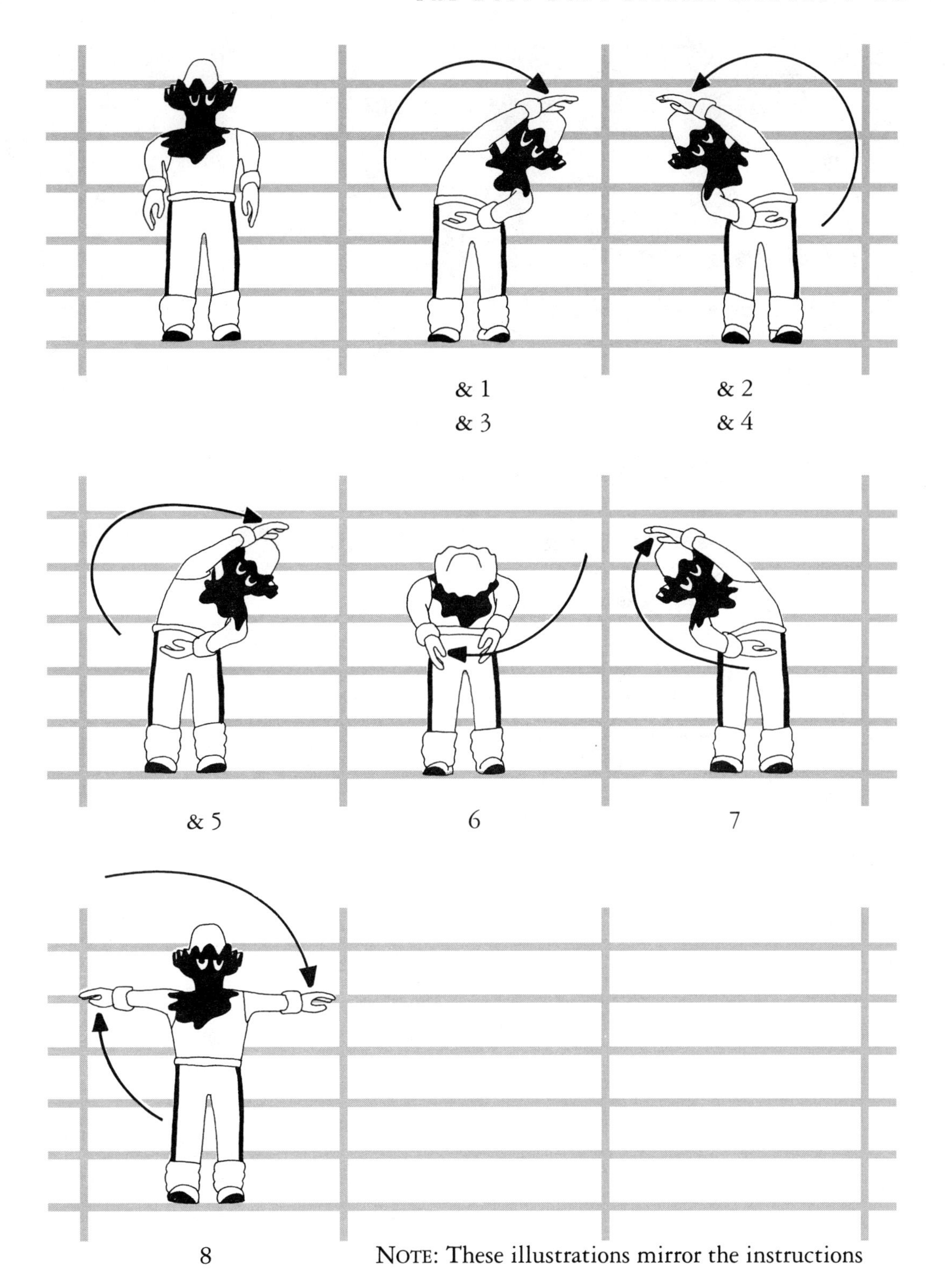

NOTE: These illustrations mirror the instructions

With backward torso rotation

The same combination of movements, with the circular path taken towards the back.

Following the *fifth* sideways arm swing (with the right over to the left side), the right hand completes a circular path with an overhead stretch *behind* you. As the right arm comes to the side at shoulder level, lift your left arm through side right. There will be a moment when both arms are extended sideways and the upper spine is stretched back. The left arm continues into a similar overhead backward reach, then over to the right before dropping in front to complete the circle with a relaxed movement.

Remember:

❖ This backward stretch may be quite a small movement depending on individual flexibility. The size of the movement is not important but it is essential to hold the waist in and firm, and to feel you are reaching back and high with the top of the head.

❖ Do not allow the head to drop back on the neck; here again the head is an extension of the spine.

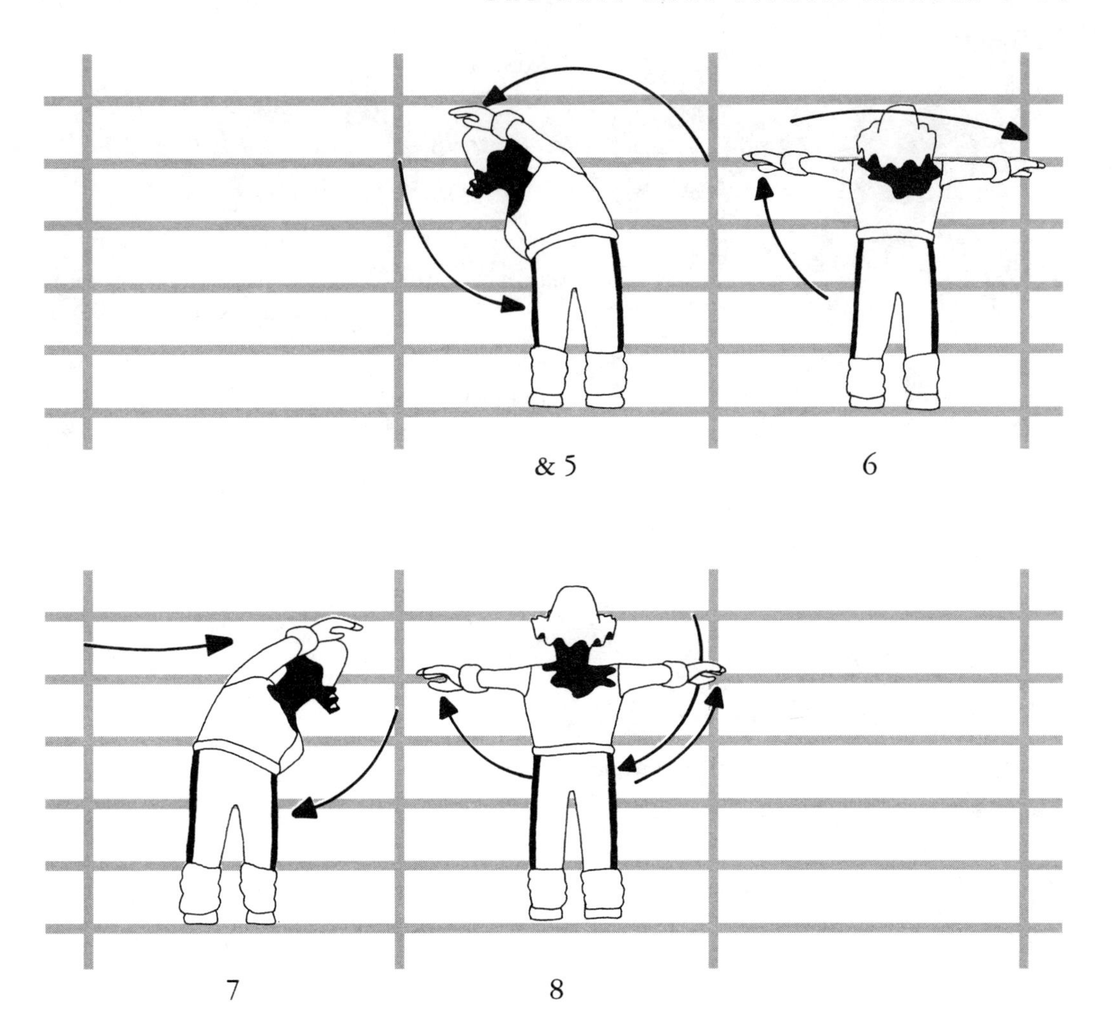
& 5
6
7
8

5 Leg swings for hip mobility

Take full advantage of gravity to diminish your effort and increase the benefit to be gained from leg swings. Practise a few swings to get the feeling.

Stand with your weight on the left leg and place the right in line behind you with your toes on the floor. Place your arms out sideways for balance. Your supporting foot may be slightly turned out for balance, but the swinging leg should maintain the forward and backward direction.

Forward and back

Brush ('brush' is the crucial term for this movement) the right foot along the floor past the left and lift the thigh and knee to a comfortable height.

& 1

Drop the right leg to allow the foot to brush past the left, carrying the thigh back and letting the lower leg fold back from the knee.

& 2

Make this forward and backward swing for a count of seven.

& 3–& 7 &

Step forwards on the right foot, transferring the weight onto it and releasing the left to repeat the whole.

8

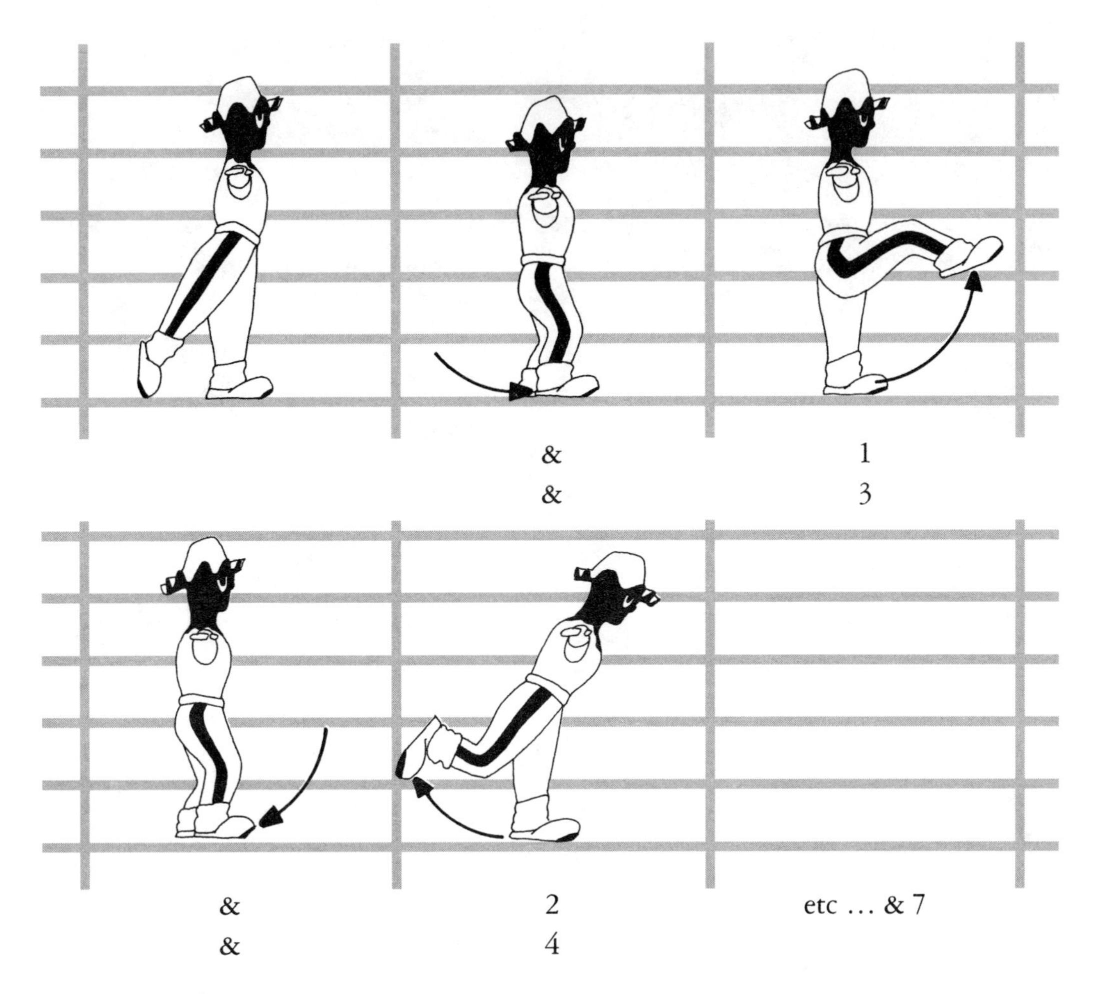

Remember:

❖ The forward and back leg swings are a simple warm-up for the hip joint. Consequently you need apply only sufficient energy to raise the thigh. Let gravity and the momentum of the swing do the rest.

❖ Allow the knee of the supporting leg to flex as the working leg drops, and to stretch (without force) as it rises.

❖ Hold the upper torso steady and the head erect to help with balance.

❖ Begin with an easy, low movement; you can increase the height and vigour of the swings later on.

❖ Balance and poise are helped by an image of being suspended by a cord from the top of the head.

Swings across the body, to the side and circling

Standing on your right foot with the left foot prepared to the side, brush the left foot along the floor in front of the right, lifting the left thigh across your centre body line.

& 1

Drop the left leg, brushing the foot on the floor as you swing the thigh into an open sideways lift.

& 2

Make an outward circular path with your knee by dropping the leg again, passing the thigh across your centre line, lifting it and carrying it out to the left.

& 3

Drop it again and lift it to the crossed position.

& A 4

Reverse this pattern by dropping the leg and swinging it out to the side, brushing across in front. Make an inward circular path by dropping the leg and lifting to the open position, lifting in front and across your centre line before dropping and brushing out sideways again.

From here you are ready to step onto the left foot to release the right for the swing and circle sequence.

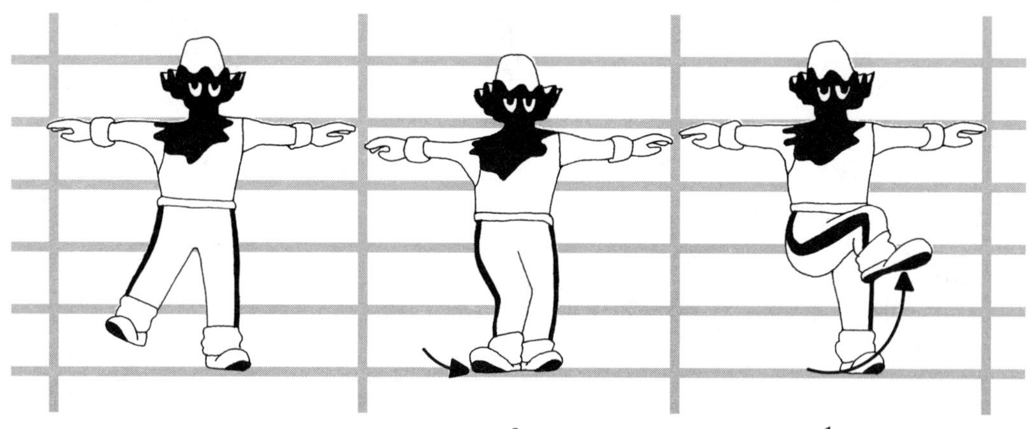

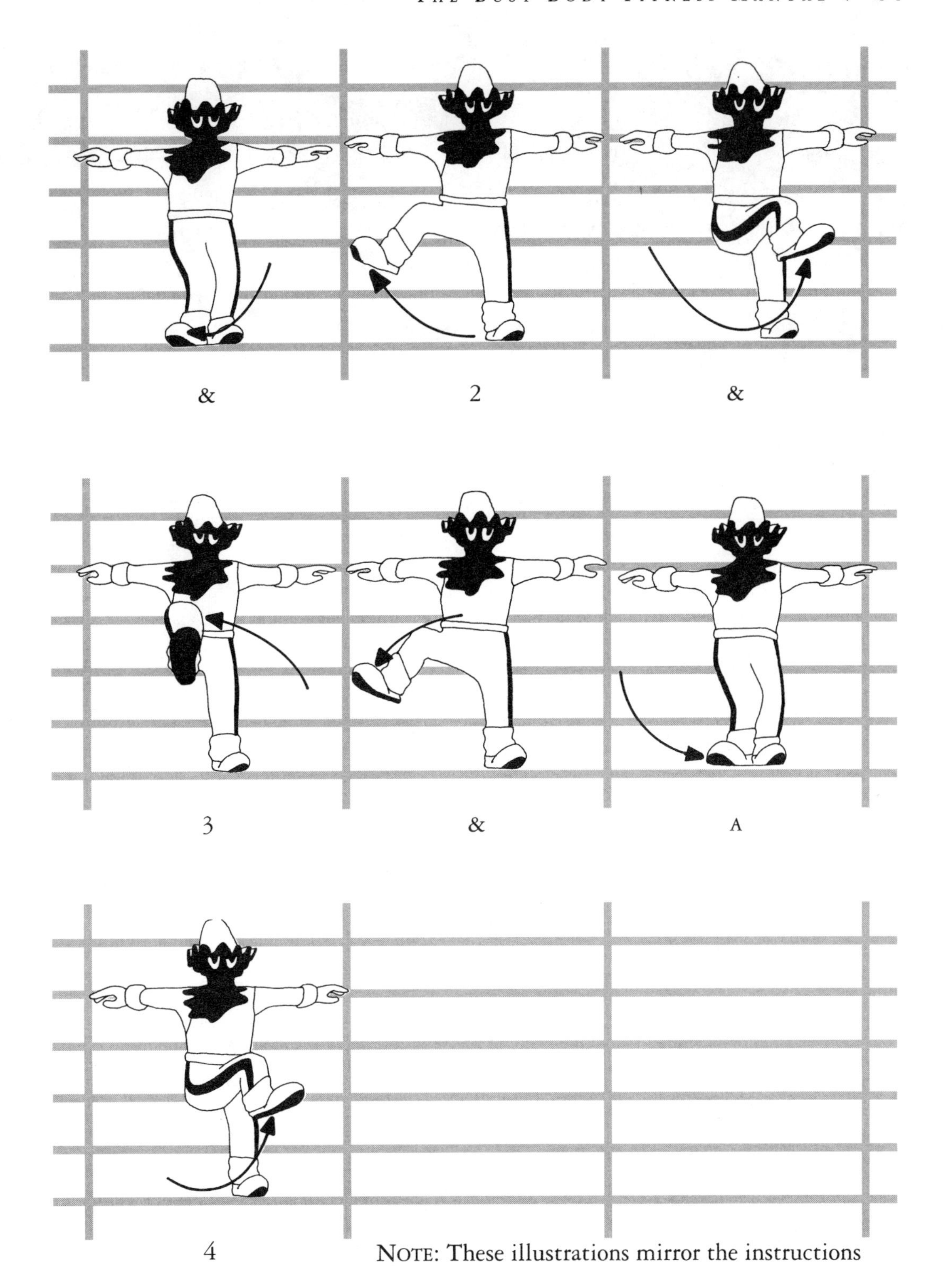

NOTE: These illustrations mirror the instructions

Remember:

❖ The side swings take advantage of gravity and momentum in the same way as the previous exercises, but require considerably more energy, especially on the circular movement. The pattern is similar to that used for arms in the first sway exercise.

❖ As for the forward and backward swings, begin with a small movement and increase the height and vigour as balance and strength permit. For better balance, keep the supporting knee flexing and stretching, hold the torso steady, focus straight ahead with the eyes, and retain the image of suspension through the top of the head.

6 Twist swing to loosen and strengthen the back

This movement is designed to maintain the full mobility of the spine.

Stand erect with shoulders and arms relaxed. The feet and hips need to be firmly anchored so you may need to place your parallel feet slightly wider apart than your hip width.

Raise your long, relaxed arms sideways to an angle of about 45° from your body and at the same time quickly turn your shoulders to face the left side and allow the arms to drop against your body; do the same quick shoulder turn to the right side. Continue to do this turn to left and right, using your shoulders as the impetus for the turn and leaving your arms relaxed; they will wrap around you further than your shoulders take them.

Flex your knees slightly as you twist, and straighten them as your arms swing out to go to the other side. Check your knees are in line over your toes; this will help keep your hips facing forwards and avoid them turning with the upper torso.

When you have experienced the twist swing, try the following combination with a roll forward and stretch back on a side diagonal turn for further flexibility in the upper spine.

Twist swing

Make eight twist swings, beginning with the right side.

1–8

Turn your shoulders—with arms stretched sideways—to face diagonally to the right forward corner; your head retains its natural alignment with your shoulders while your hips remain facing the front in alignment with your feet.

COUNT 1 FOR THE TURN AND HOLD FOR COUNT 2

Drop your arms and roll forward with head and torso as far as possible without releasing below the waist.

3, 4

Unroll and raise your arms sideways to a high V shape, with your head reaching back and chest fully stretched.

5, 6

Swing your arms into an inwards circle across your body, out to the sides, and let them drop as you turn your shoulders to face the front to repeat the whole movement, beginning on the left.

7, 8

Remember:

❖ This exercise uses the spine's vertical mobility to the full. Maximise the twist by looking behind you with each turn.

❖ Ensure that your feet and hips are well anchored and don't allow them to turn with your upper body.

❖ Check that your shoulders are remaining perpendicular to your spine and that you are not including a sideways or forwards bend in your twist.

❖ The roll forwards and reach back may be small movements: that is not important. The focus is on maintaining your personal level of mobility.

❖ The extent of the sideways turn will also depend on your flexibility; check that you are not compensating with sideways distortion or by releasing the hips.

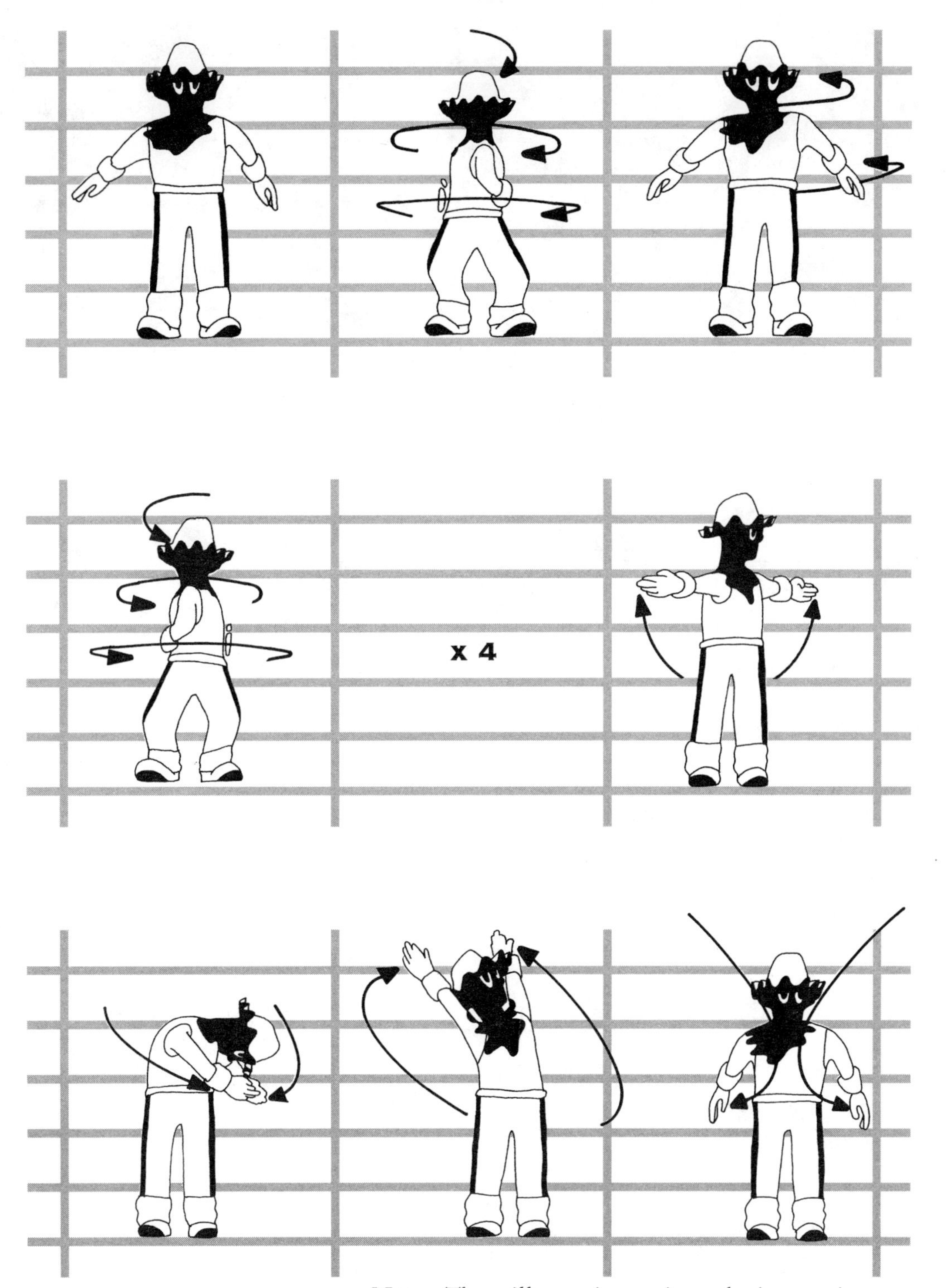

NOTE: These illustrations mirror the instructions

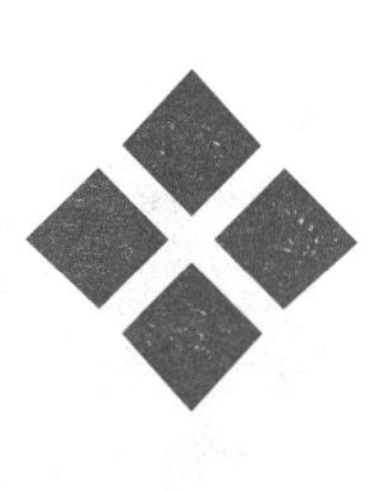

7 *Arm circling with walks, forward body curve and balance*

This is a 'quickie' to serve as an invigorator whenever you have a couple of minutes between jobs or while you're waiting for the kettle to boil. Here the word 'step' means a walking step; transfer your weight wholly on each of the first four counts.

Arm circles and roll — a two minute quickie

Stepping right foot forward, swing both arms forward then raise them high and circle them out and down.

1 &

Stepping left foot forward, swing both arms forward and up and look up. Hold for a moment before reversing with the next step.

2 &

Stepping right foot back, swing both arms forward and down, then circle out and up.

3 &

Stepping left foot back, swing both arms forward and down, then circle out and up.

4

Place your right foot parallel with your left to continue the arms' circle, taking your torso in a forward curve as your arms reach back behind, at the same time as your knees flex and stretch.

& 5

Reverse the circle with your arms (repeating the knee flex and stretch) to raise your torso.

& 6

Pause with arms high and lift your weight onto the balls of your feet, achieving a balance.

& 7, & 8

Repeat the sequence, beginning with the left foot.

Remember:

❖ The whole combination should be done with a feeling of lightness and suspension, especially on the final balance. It may take a few repeats to achieve that sensation.

❖ On the forward curve, give a soft bounce and stretch through the knees on & 5 and another on & 6 to maintain a relaxed swing through the sequence.

❖ The forward curve here involves the same principle as the roll explained at length for Exercise 2. That is, the long curve of the spine is achieved by tucking the hips under, lifting the navel, and letting the head relax forward.

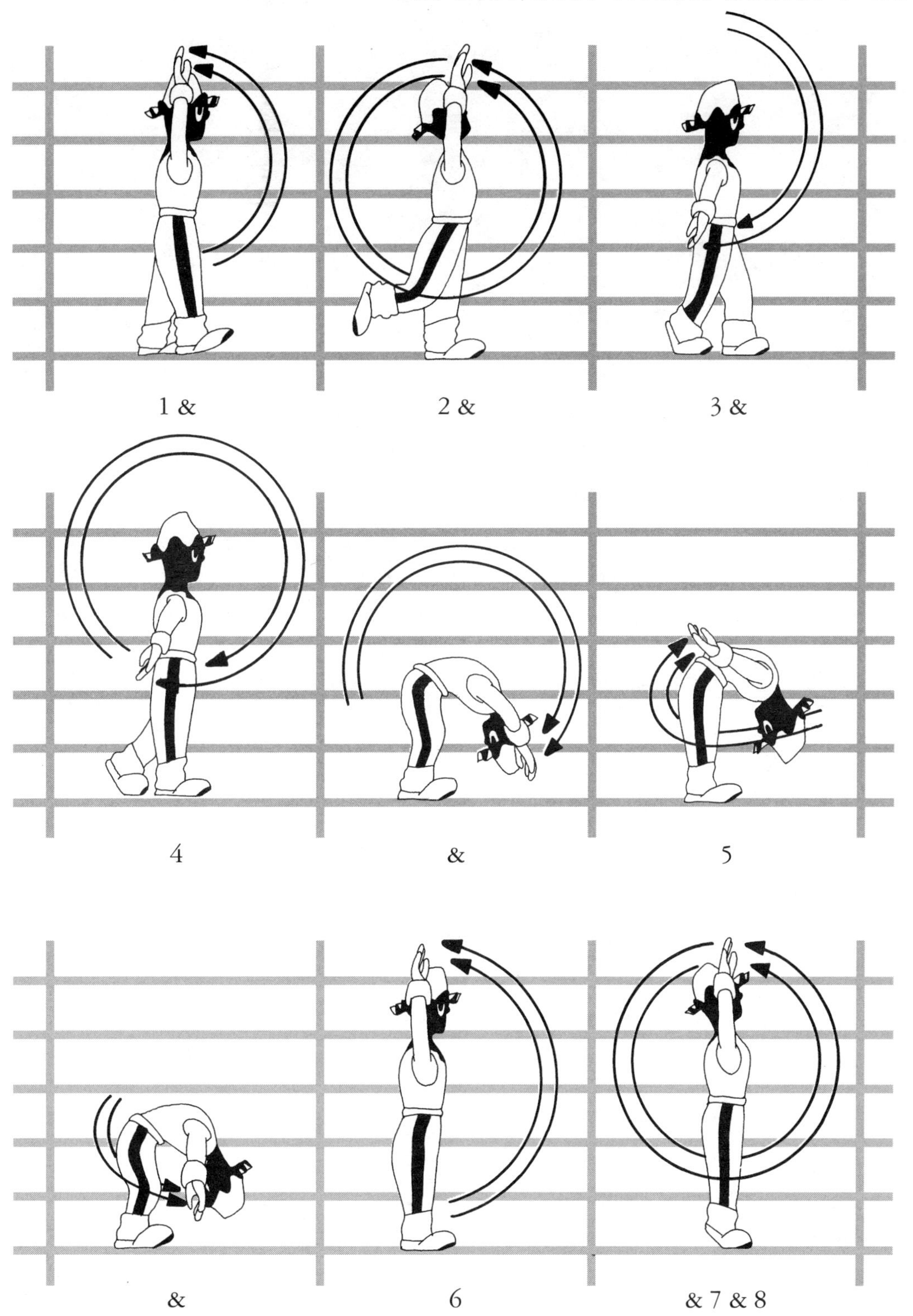
1 &
2 &
3 &
4
&
5
&
6
& 7 & 8

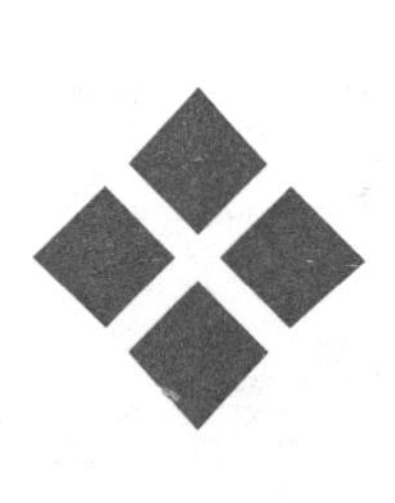

Floor SEQUENCES

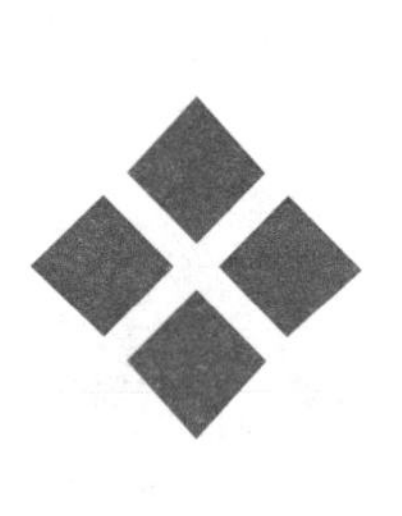

Full stretch

Floor exercises are designed to relax the joints (especially hips and shoulders, since body weight is more evenly distributed in the horizontal position), to strengthen the abdomen while taking care of the spine, and to tone up the legs.

Begin by lying on your back, legs slightly apart and arms likewise above your head, and stretching to your maximum in both directions.

Relax, placing your arms just away from your sides and your legs together. Consider how much of your spine is in contact with the floor. For most people, an area in the small of the back (near the waistline) and the neck will not touch.

Bend your knees, placing the soles of your feet against the floor about 30 cm distant from your sitting bones.

From this position bring the whole length of the spine in contact with the floor. This may need a conscious effort for the small of the back, and you will find there is a spot at the base of the skull where it is impossible; raise your head slightly and as you replace it, think of putting the vertebrae as near to the floor as you can to achieve maximum length. From here you can roll your head from side to side on the floor to feel more relaxed.

There are various movements, designed to work on the abdomen, that start from a position lying on your back and lifting either or both ends of your body. This can put a great strain on the back unless certain safety criteria are observed.

Begin by establishing firm contact with the floor with the whole of your spine and especially the back of the waist.

When you have your spine fully in contact with the floor, slowly peel the lower vertebrae away one by one so that the hips tilt up/under, and then replace them in reverse sequence. It is essential to experience this position because many movements rely on it both when exercising the abdomen and to safeguard the lower and middle spine. As you tilt the base of your spine away from the floor, consciously contract and flatten your abdominal muscles. Become familiar with this contracting action so that you can bring it into play when required.

Holding the hip-tilt and contraction, raise your head and shoulders slightly, reaching with your fingertips past your thighs and knees, trying to maintain the flat abdomen. This may seem impossible at first but will gradually be achieved by focusing on that goal whenever you do this work. You can refer to the illustrations for sequence 9 for this movement.

A FINAL NOTE: An important point to observe is *never to lift both legs at once*: always hold one leg bent with the foot anchoring your hips against the floor, or have one knee bent into your body and maintain the contact between the spine and the floor.

8 *Half and whole maxi circles with the leg*

I use this exercise to loosen and relax my hip joints, lumbar region and lower spine. It's best to take it gently for the first half-dozen moves and, as it feels looser and easier, progress to the combination which includes the leg opening to the side and the complete circle.

PREPARATION

Lie on your back, legs parallel and knees bent, and arms out sideways for stability.

Stretch your right leg along the floor then draw a line on the floor with the inside of that foot towards the left hand, letting the left leg (still bent) drop down sideways to the floor. The right leg, straight to begin with, will cross over the left. Allow it to bend at the knee, if necessary, and relax it so that the right foot stays in contact with the floor as it travels as near as is comfortable towards the left hand.

At this point both your shoulders will ideally still be in contact with the floor. If the right one has come away, be conscious of it and gradually relax it into the floor to achieve maximum stretch.

Retrace the path with the right foot to your centre line — making sure as you do so that the lower spine and back waistline make contact with the floor as soon as possible — and finally bend the right knee to replace the right foot beside the left. Now you are ready to do the same with the left leg.

If I decide to begin with the floor work and this is the first exercise in my fifteen minute session, I usually do this basic movement quite slowly several times on each side before proceeding to the following sequence at a nippy tempo.

Leg half and whole circles to loosen pelvis and back

From lying on your back, both knees bent and arms sideways, straighten your right leg. Draw a line on the floor with the right foot, moving it towards your left hand.

1 &, A 2

Make the right foot retrace its path to the centre line, then swing your leg out strongly sideways* to the right, foot flexed allowing the leg to lift off the floor. Anchor your hips squarely by leaving the left leg in an open position with the left foot firmly planted against the floor.

3 &, A 4

Return the straight right leg to the centre line to repeat this half circle twice more.

5–8; 1–4

Follow by bringing the straight right leg down to the centre line, across to the left, up over in front, open out to the right side again and back to centre, in a full circle.

5, 6, 7

Complete by folding the right knee up to your chest before replacing it beside the left.

&, 8

Repeat the whole sequence with the left leg.

Remember:

❖ There is a marked difference in the kind of energy you apply to the initial relaxed movement and the control and vigour necessary to hold your whole back against the floor as you swing your fully extended leg to the side. In the first movement, give in to gravity and use the weight of the leg to loosen the joints. In the second movement the straight leg gives a firm stretch to the side. (*The exact position intended by the term 'side' in this context will vary according to individual flexibility; move your leg as far to the side as physical limitations allow while keeping the lumbar region against the floor.) Stretch the working leg also on the final circle and feel the back, especially the lumbar region, squarely against the floor.

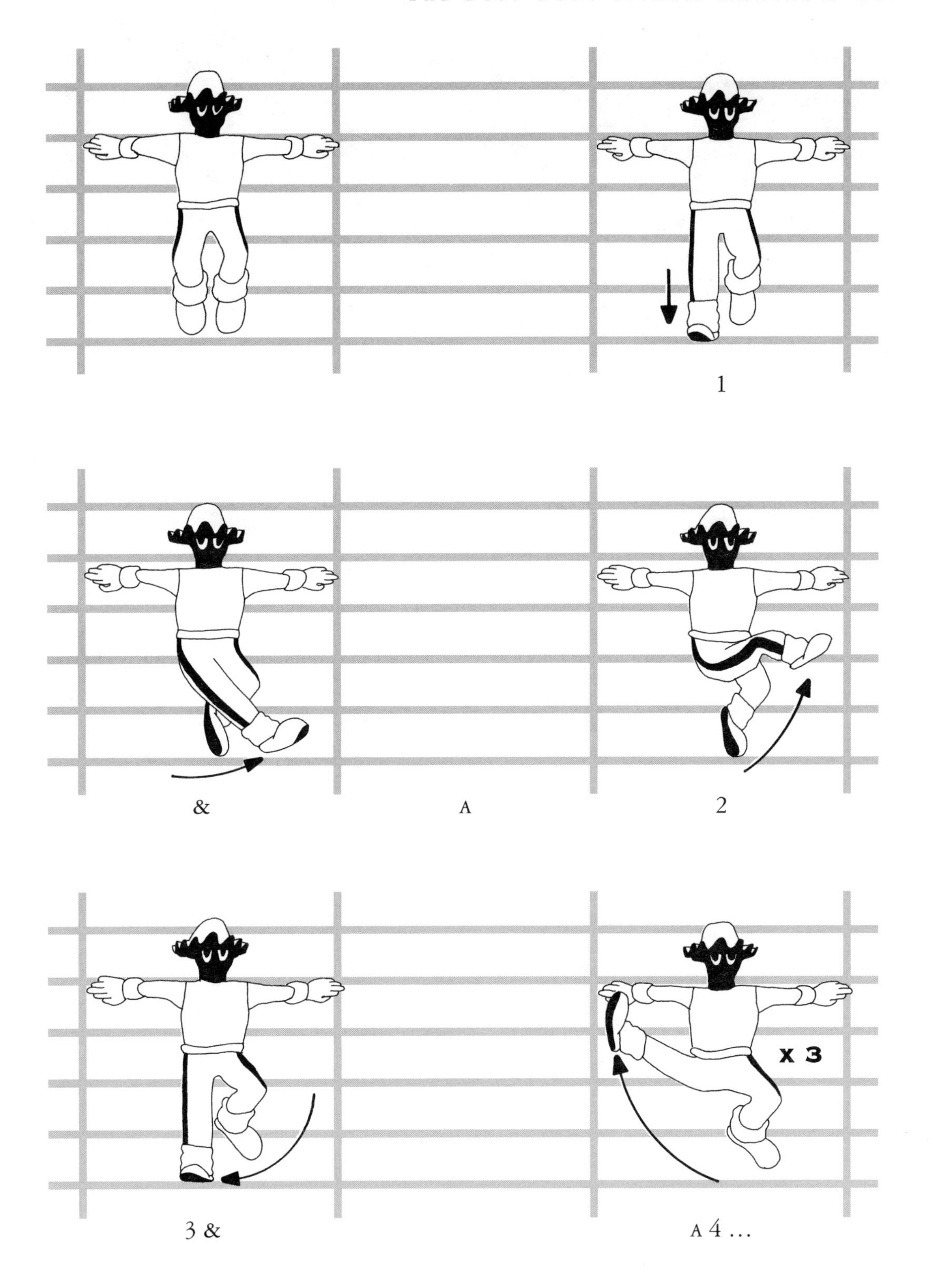
1
&
A
2
x 3
3 &
A 4 . . .

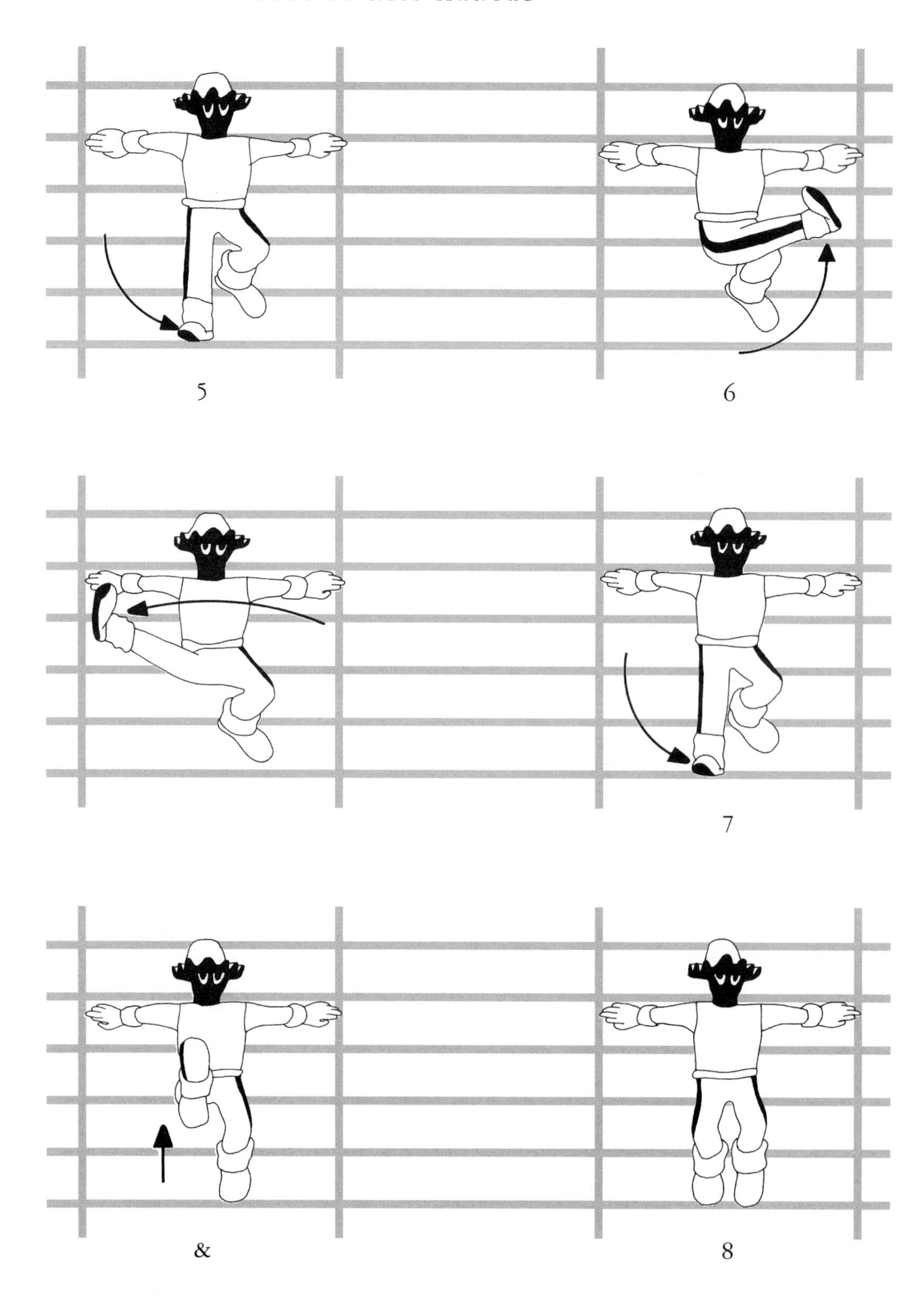
5
6
7
&
8

9 *Roll up and roll down for abdomen and back*

Lie on your back, knees bent and feet firmly planted on the floor, with your arms by your sides.

This exercise is possibly the one most commonly used to work the abdominal muscles. To obtain maximum benefit keep in mind the points stressed throughout this manual: with your spine in full contact with the floor, tilt your hips so that the lower two vertebrae come away from the floor before you attempt to raise your head and shoulders. Press your knees firmly together: you may want to place a small, soft object between your knees to maintain this pressure. Concentrate on holding the abdominal muscles as flat as possible as you roll up and down. This may seem impossible at first but will gradually happen with perseverance. Feel each vertebra returning to the floor as you go down.

Roll up and roll down

Lift your head and roll up, reaching with your fingers just beyond your bent knees.

1, 2

Return to lie on the floor.

3, 4

Repeat.

5–8

Roll up a third time.

1, 2

Push forward with the lower spine to sit upright as you stretch your legs along the floor and move your arms forward and raise above your head.

& 3

Open your arms sideways, looking upwards.

4

Pull your navel inwards and tilt your hips forward to initiate an even roll down, ready to repeat the whole sequence.

5–8

Remember:

❖ Keep an even flow throughout and avoid jerks.

❖ Facilitate the smoothness of the roll back to the floor by bringing your arms and head forward to act as a counterbalance.

❖ As you roll down to begin again, see how long you can keep your legs straight with your spine in contact with the floor. They will probably need to bend just before you complete the roll.

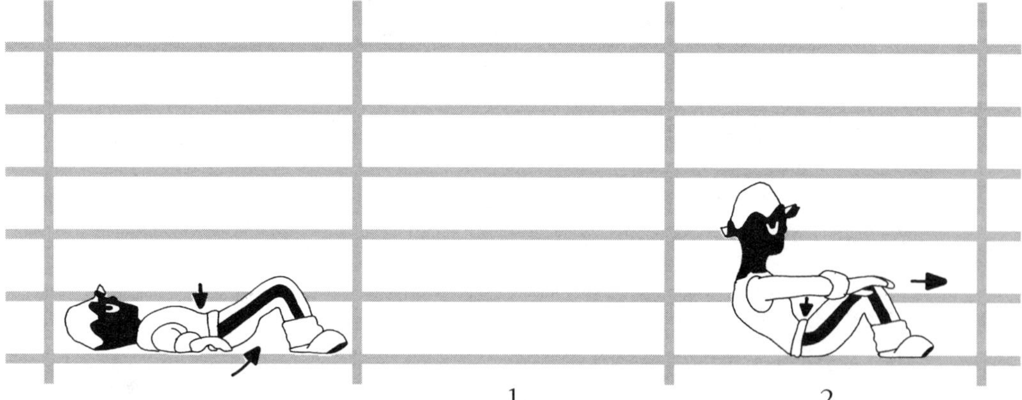

1…
5

2
6

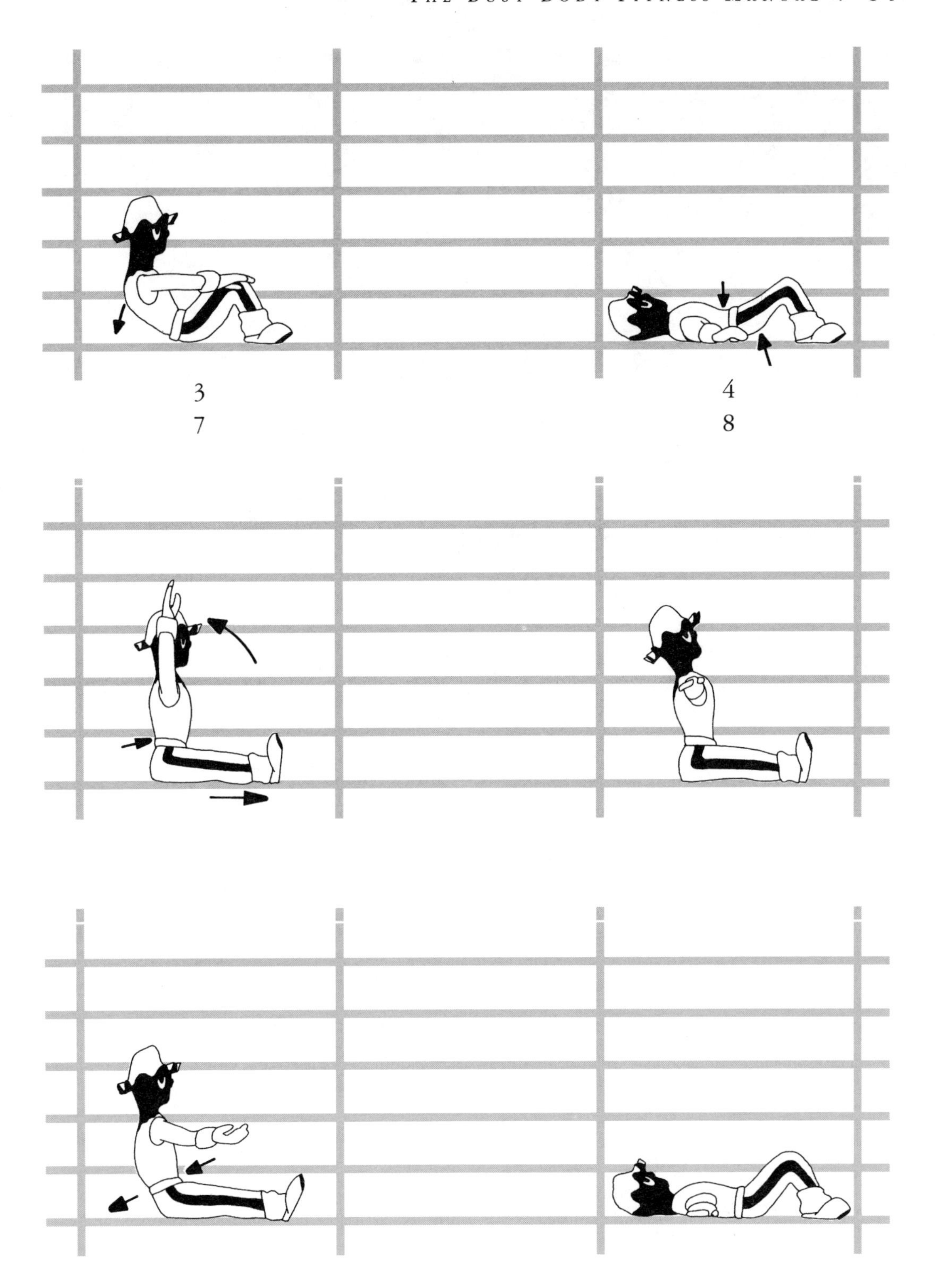
3
7
4
8

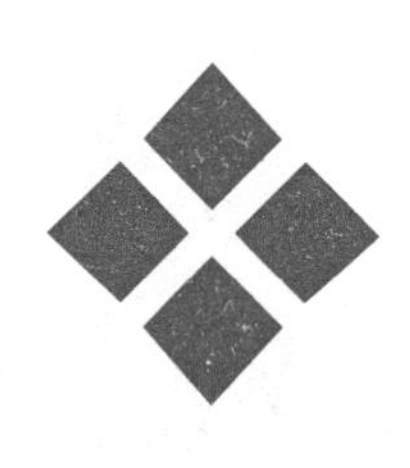

10

Mini circles and stirring for the hip joint

Lie on your back with your left leg bent and foot firmly planted on the floor, and the right leg straight and slightly off the floor. Both legs are comfortably turned out from the hip, and the spine (especially at the waist) is pressed into the floor. Arms are out sideways for stability. The outward and inward mini circles work the thigh and lower abdomen muscles as long as you hold your spine against the floor.

The stirring movement is a mobility exercise for the hip joint: the heel follows a circular path as a consequence of your thigh rotation as though you were stirring a large cauldron. To stir, draw your right knee up sideways in the turned out position giving maximum fold in the hip socket; bring the right knee in front of the chest, then stretch the leg down (still raised) in line with your centre, and slightly outwards to repeat.

Mini leg circles and stir

Draw eight small outward circles with your straight right leg.

1–8

Draw eight small inward circles with your straight right leg.

1–8

Stir six times with the right heel, finishing with heels together.

1–8 AND 1–4

Push both feet along the floor until the legs are straight.

5, 6

Bend the right leg, placing your foot firmly on the floor.

7

Raise the left leg slightly to repeat the sequence with the left leg.

8

Remember:

❖ Keep ankles flexed for a stronger movement and maintain turnout.

❖ Maintain contact between your spine and the floor. Your back at the waistline may come away from the floor as you stretch both legs. Make sure you replace it as you prepare to repeat.

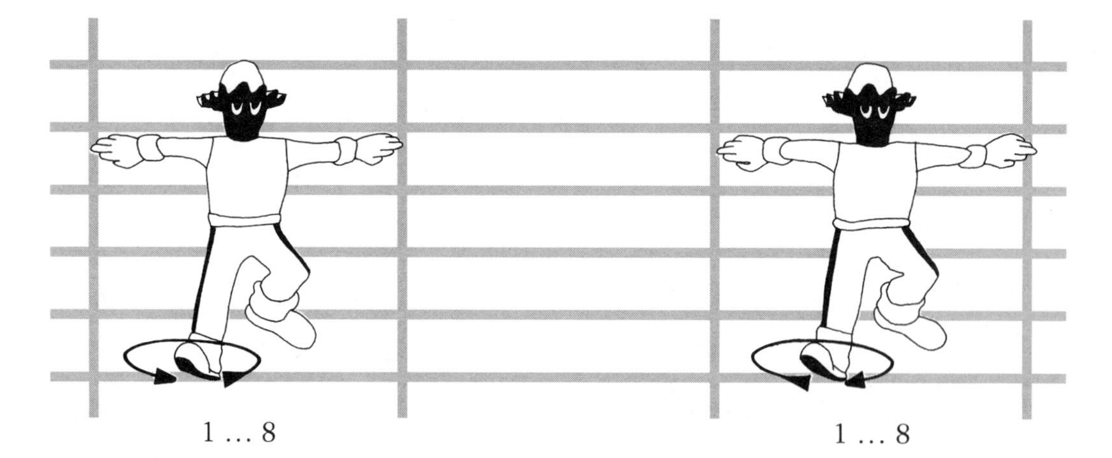

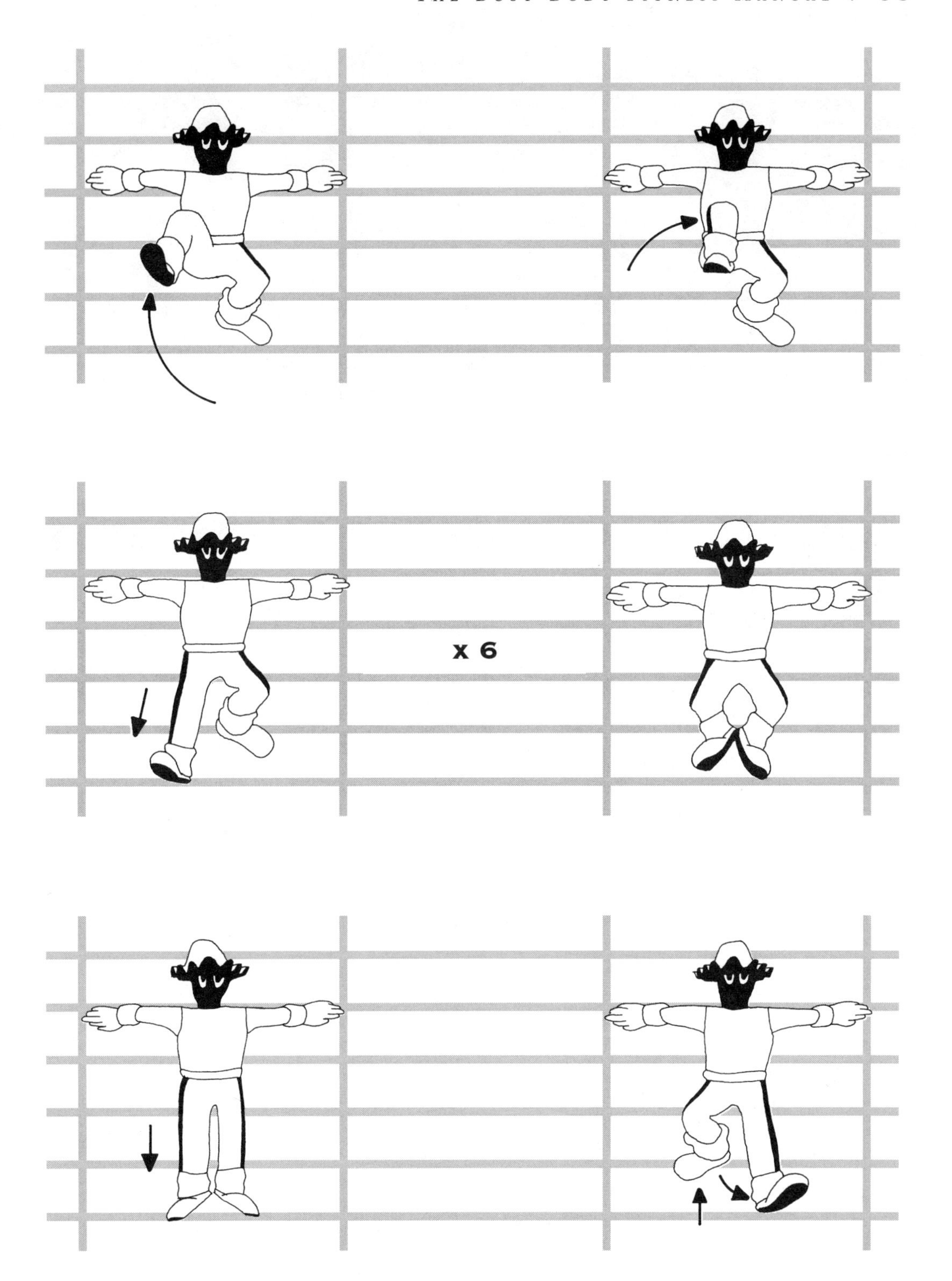
x 6

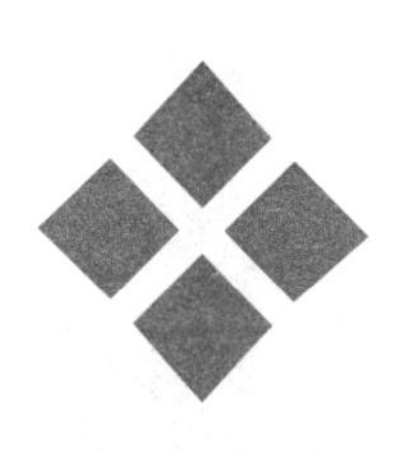

11 *Raising shoulders and leg to strengthen abdomen*

Lie on your back, knees bent and feet firmly planted against the floor. Stretch your left leg at the same time as you raise your head and shoulders, and bring your right knee towards the right shoulder, grasping the right shin with both hands. This is easier if the right hand is near the ankle and the left just below the knee.

Check your middle spine is in contact with the floor and abdomen contracted as you hold this position briefly then relax and repeat with the other leg. Try this several times before combining with backwards cycling movements.

Raising shoulders and leg simultaneously, followed with cycling

Raise head and shoulders and grasp your right shin as you stretch your left leg.

1

Hold the position.

2

Relax back slightly, bringing your left knee beside the right and releasing your grasp.

3, 4

Repeat all with the other leg.

5–8

Repeat the whole sequence again (four times in all).

1–8

Return your shoulders and head to the floor and do four backward cycling leg movements in slow counts.

1–8

Follow with eight double-time backward cycling movements.

1–8

Remember:

- Focus on holding your middle spine in contact with the floor throughout.
- For the cycling movement, the nearer your leg comes to achieving a line parallel to the floor when it is straight, the more you work the abdominal muscles. This needs to be balanced by well-folded thigh and knee joints on the other leg and a well-controlled flat abdomen. Check that your neck is relaxed and breathe easily.

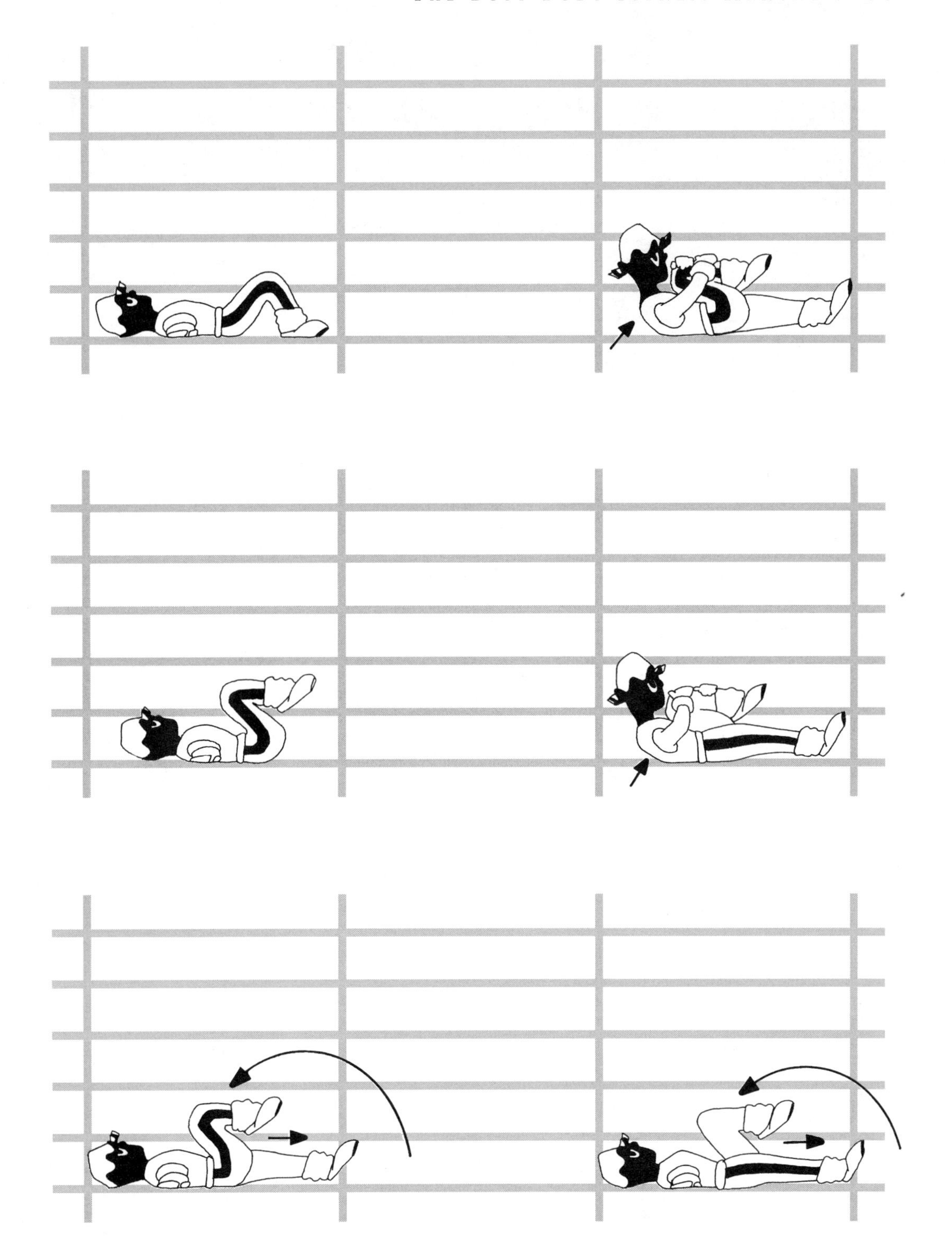

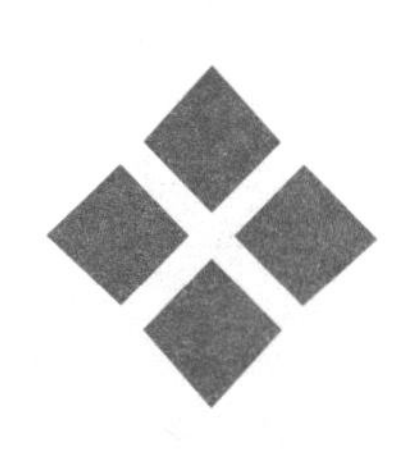

12

Contract, extend and tilt for upper back strength

This sequence has two parts. For the first, sit on the floor with knees bent and open, and the soles of your feet together; the movement works the torso in line with the hips. For the second, sit with legs stretched apart; the movement works the torso on a diagonal to the hips. The torso contraction with forward roll, followed by the stretch into a flat back, may be quite small. Again the focus is on activating the relevant parts. The side stretch uses the arms to define the direction of the tilt, and gives added strength to the back as well as flexibility.

FIRST PART

Start from the sitting position, hands resting on the knees, spine held erect and head easily balanced. Then make the following moves using two counts for each position.

❖ Pull your navel in towards your spine, pushing back at your waist and tilting the hips under. At the same time drop your head forward to increase the length and curve of your spine as far as you can without slumping.

❖ Push forward with the top of your head, pulling your back into a long flat line.

❖ Return to the erect position by reaching forward with your arms and then raising them above your head.

❖ Open your arms to the side at shoulder height with palms upwards and reach high and back with your head to fully extend the erect spine.

❖ Tilt your torso sideways right from the waist (maintaining the relationship of arms and head to shoulders) until the fingers and back of the right hand touch the floor.

❖ Allow your right elbow to bend so that your weight is taken onto your forearm and reach overhead to the right with your left (straight) arm to a full side stretch. (Check your left buttock is still anchored to the floor; if it is not, aim to replace it.)

❖ Recover your erect position, returning your left arm and extending the right as you straighten. You may need to push away from the floor with your right arm initially until you gain strength.

❖ Repeat the sideways tilt to the left side and recover to repeat the whole.

On the straight

Contract and curve forward.

1 & 2

Stretch to a flat back position.

3 & 4

Return to sitting erect, with arms held high.

5 & 6

Open your arms to the side, palms upwards, and look up.

7 & 8

Tilt sideways to the right, reaching over with your left arm.

1 & 2

Return torso to the erect position.

3 & 4

Repeat the tilt on the left side.

5 & 6

Return to the erect position and replace your hands in their original position. Repeat the whole sequence.

7 & 8

Remember:

❖ Sitting erect in the initial position will probably feel as though you are leaning back. In a natural, relaxed position your body will lean forward from the hips. Although the counts 1–4 movement is quite small, it brings muscles of the back well into play. During the counts 5–8 section, your shoulders must be relaxed down (not tense and hunched). As you reach back with your head on 7 and 8, retain a long neck (do not allow your head to drop back to break the neck line). Aim to keep the side tilt in one plane, without any twist. If the position feels awkward initially, remain in the position with your weight on your forearm; it will gradually feel more comfortable.

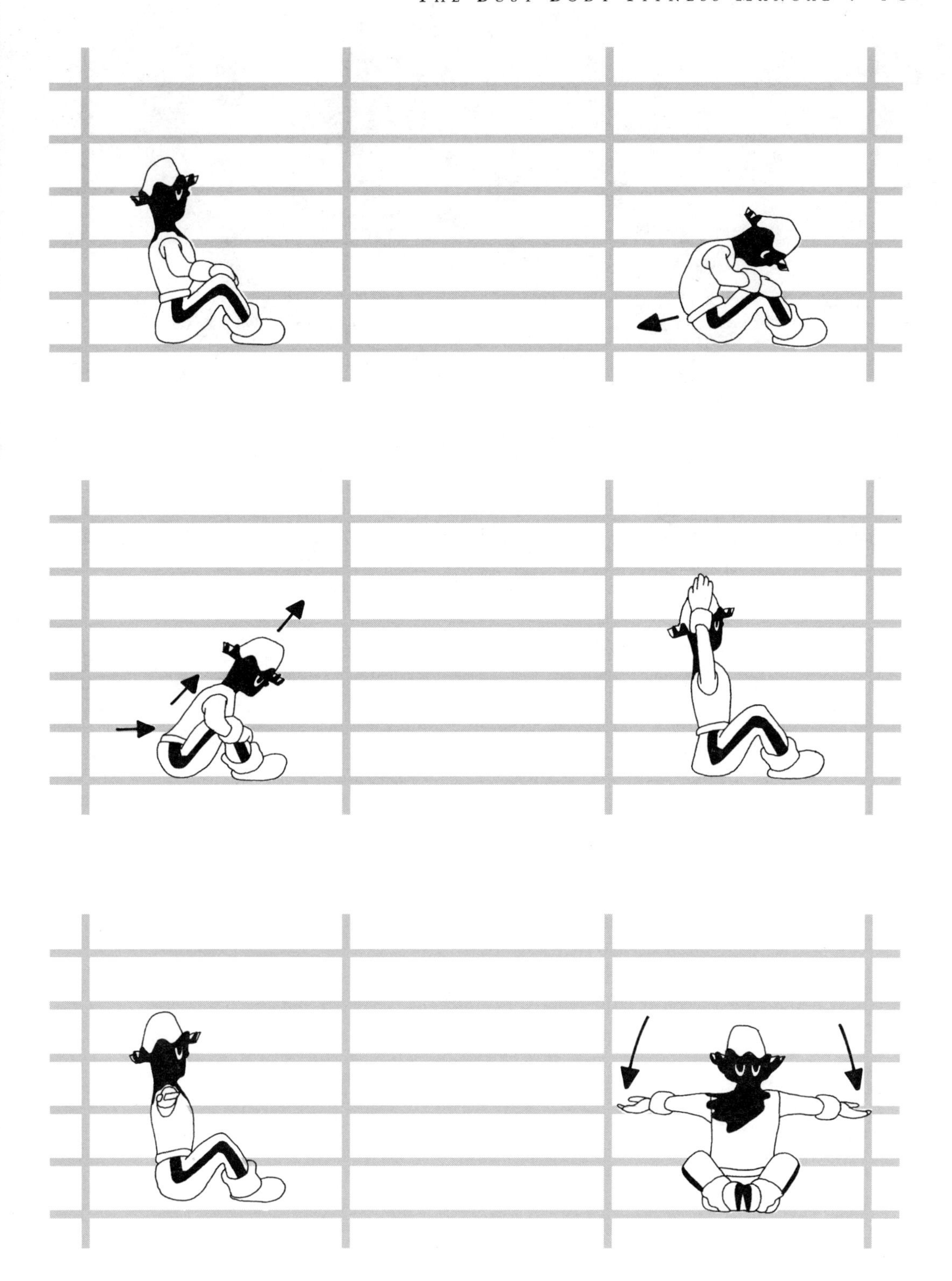

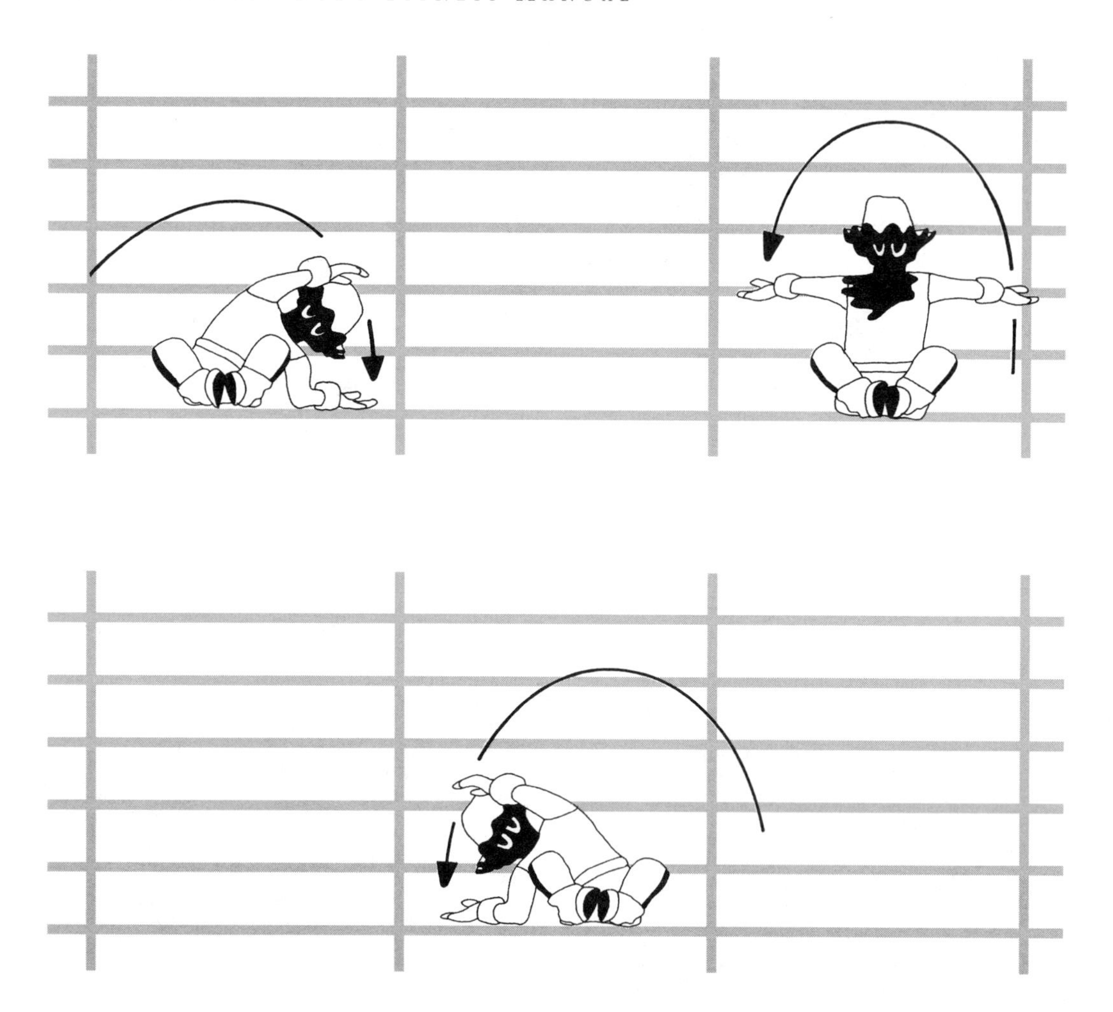

SECOND PART

The sequence of movements is basically the same as for the first part except that it is taken from a sitting position with the legs straight and opened as far as is comfortably possible. Sit tall and turn your upper torso so that you are facing the direction of your left leg; place your hands easily on the floor on either side of your left thigh.

❖ On the first contraction your head goes down towards your left knee.

❖ As you push forwards with the top of your head to flatten your back, your torso stretch will be in the same direction as your leg.

❖ Maintain this direction as you stretch your arms forward and lift them above your head.

❖ As you open your arms sideways to shoulder level, look towards your left hand.

❖ For the first sideways tilt go to the left, putting the left forearm on the floor and taking the right arm overhead to make the side stretch. The second sideways tilt goes along the right leg with the left arm overhead.

On the diagonal

Contract and curve your torso, moving your head towards your left knee.

1, 2

Push forward with your head into a flat back position.

3, 4

Reach forward with your hands then raise your arms above your head.

5, 6

Open the arms to shoulder level, looking towards the left hand.

7, 8

Tilt your torso sideways left to rest on your left forearm.

1, 2

Return torso to erect position.

3, 4

Tilt torso sideways right along the direction of your right leg stretching over with the left arm.

5, 6

Return torso to erect position.

7, 8

Remember:

❖ As you reach forward and raise your arms on counts 5 and 6, be conscious of your long, erect spine and balanced head. Although the movements are again quite small, this exercise is very effective in strengthening and maintaining the line of the upper torso and, as a consequence, counteracting the tendency to stoop.

❖ Check the clear sideways plane of your side bends; avoid relaxing into a forward bend.

❖ Keep your shoulders relaxed, not tense and hunched.

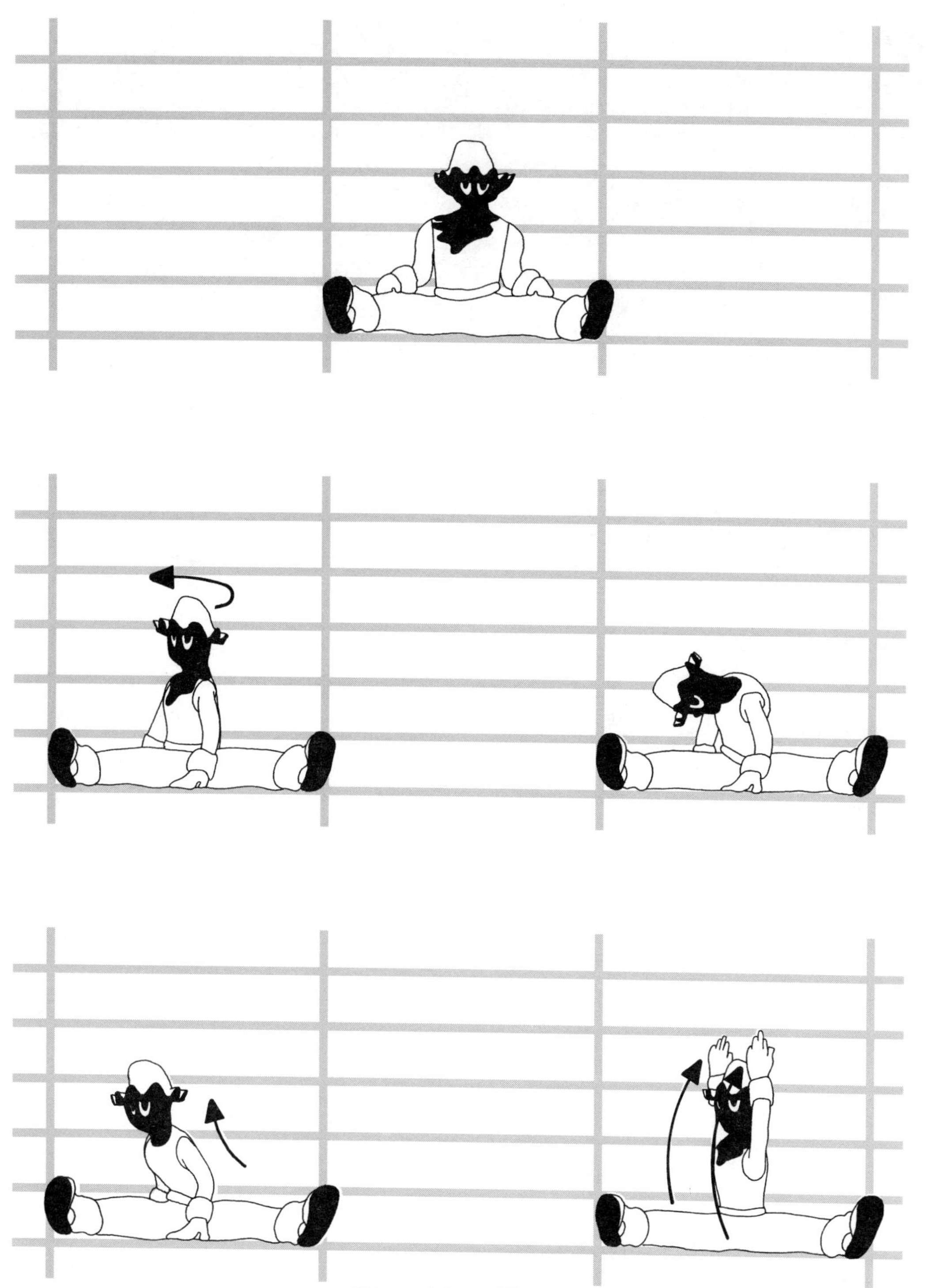

NOTE: These illustrations mirror the instructions

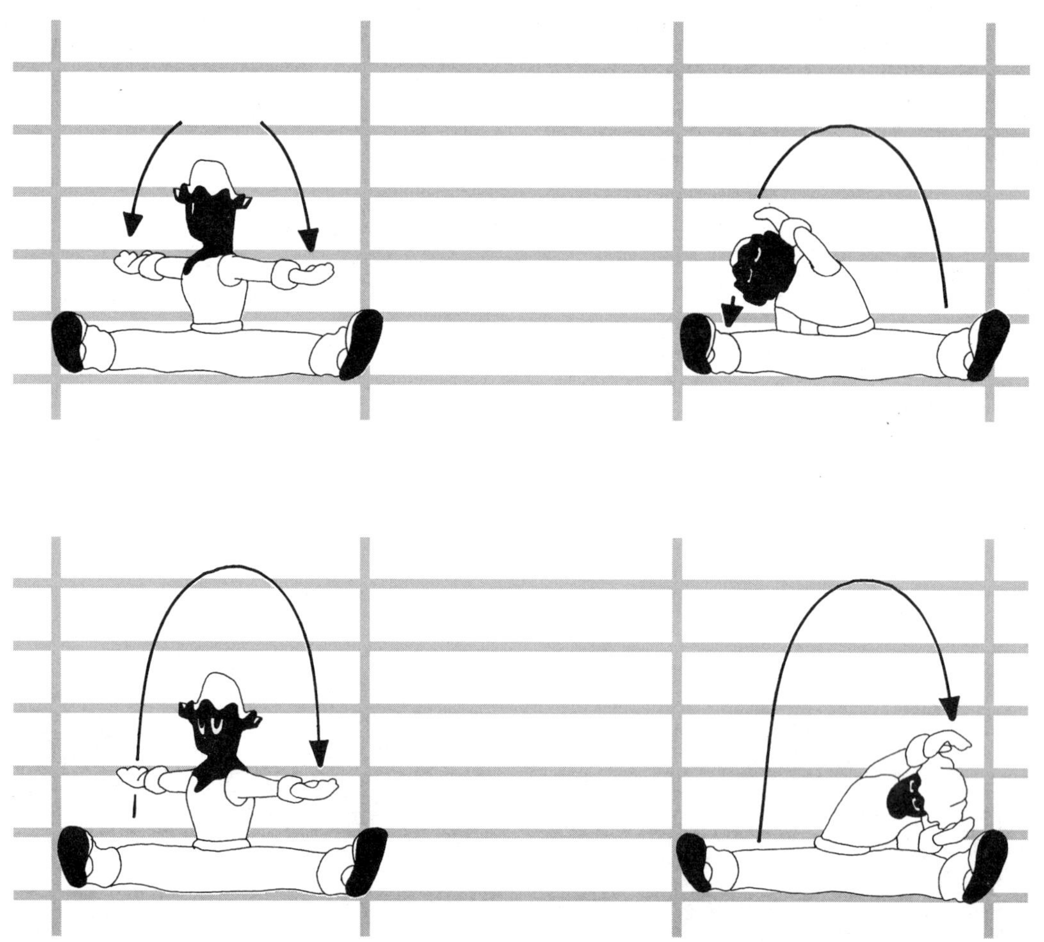

NOTE: These illustrations mirror the instructions

Final stretch

Finish your session with a stretch lying on your front.

From this prone position choose one or more of the following:

❖ Place your hands near your shoulders to lift one long straight leg and then the other.

❖ Lift one arm and the opposite leg at the same time, maintaining maximum length from fingertips to stretched toes.

❖ For a good stretch lift both arms and legs together, then think of holding the muscles of the abdomen as well as stretching in both directions.

❖ Place your hands near your shoulders to raise the head and upper torso. This yoga position, the Cobra, is excellent to end with.

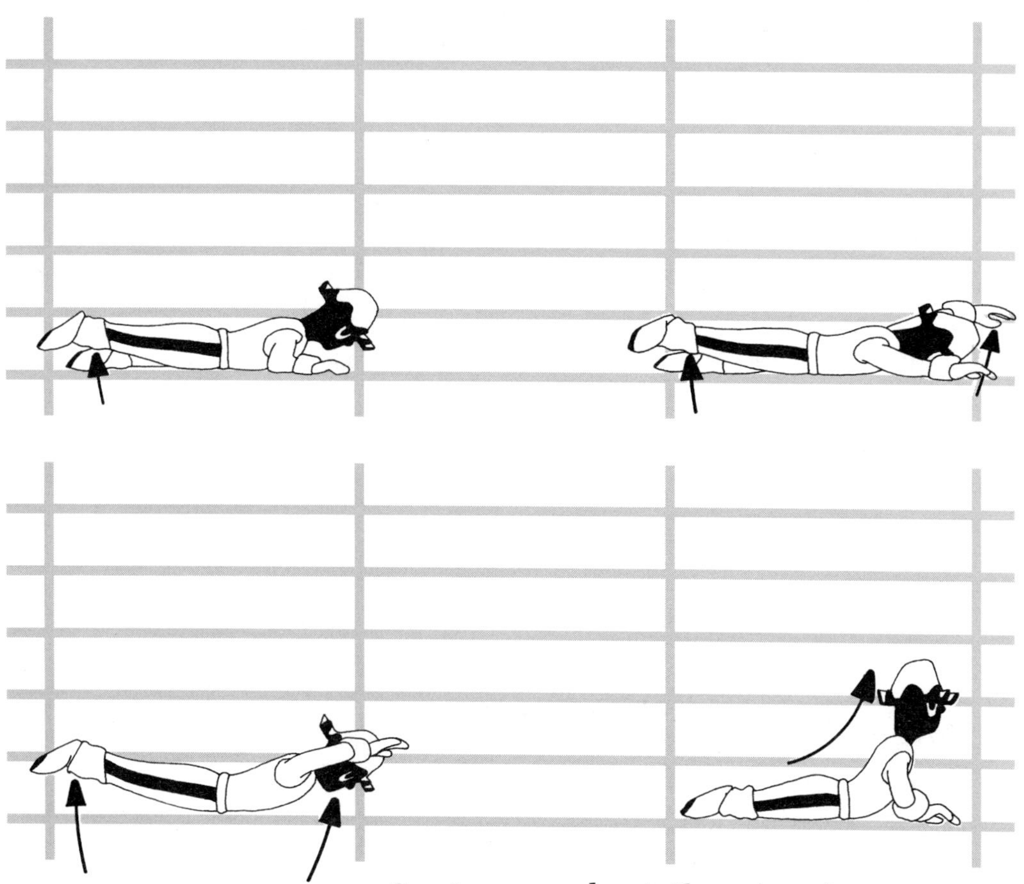

Session complete! Come again tomorrow.

Suggestions for accompanying music

Suggestions for music to accompany the sequences have been selected from amongst the wealth of recordings of Thomas 'Fats' Waller.

SONG TITLE	SEQUENCE REFERENCE
My Very Good Friend The Milkman	1. Sways 2. Reach and roll 5. Leg swings 6. Twist swings
I'm Gonna Sit Right Down And Write Myself A Letter	7. Arm circling 8. Half and whole leg circles
Baby Brown	1. Sways 2. Reach and roll 4. Side bends
Whose Honey Are You	3. Leg lift 4. Side bends
Blue Because Of You	8. Half and whole leg circles 9. Roll up and down
You've Been Taking Lessons In Love	10. Mini leg circles 11. Raise leg and shoulders
Just As Long As The World Goes Round and Round	5. Leg swings 10. Mini leg circles
I'm On A Seesaw	5. Leg swings 6. Twist swings
Sweet Thing	12. Contract, extend and tilt
Rhythm And Romance	4. Side bends (at slower tempo) 10. Mini leg circles (faster tempo)

All the above tracks are included in a compilation entitled 'Fats At His Finest' available on CD from Parade. This album features several other tracks that will doubtless move you to arrange your own sequences if you enjoy Fats' rhythm and humour as we do.

P. C. and G. S.